COP
AUTHOR
LAW
AUTHORSHIP
GUIDELINES
IDENTIFICATION
WEB
ADDRESS

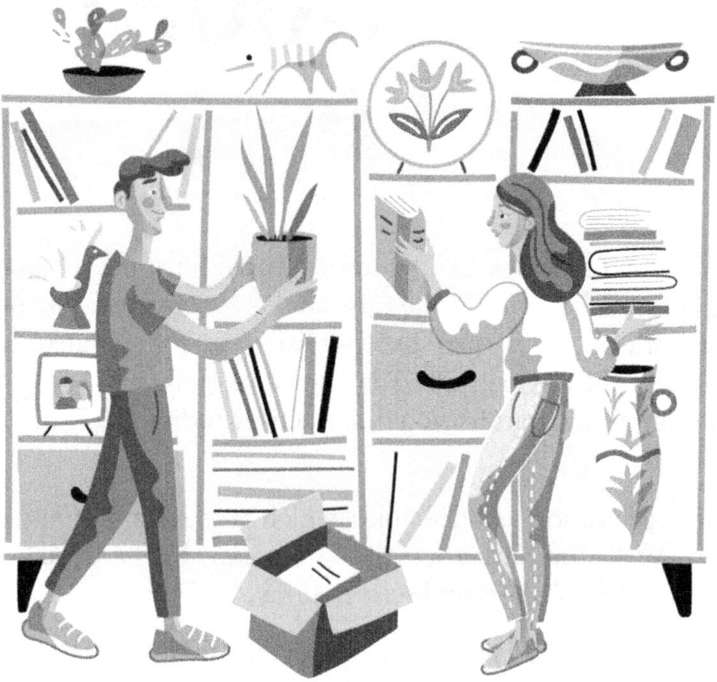

CERTIFICATE OF PREGNANCY

Due date

Table of Contents

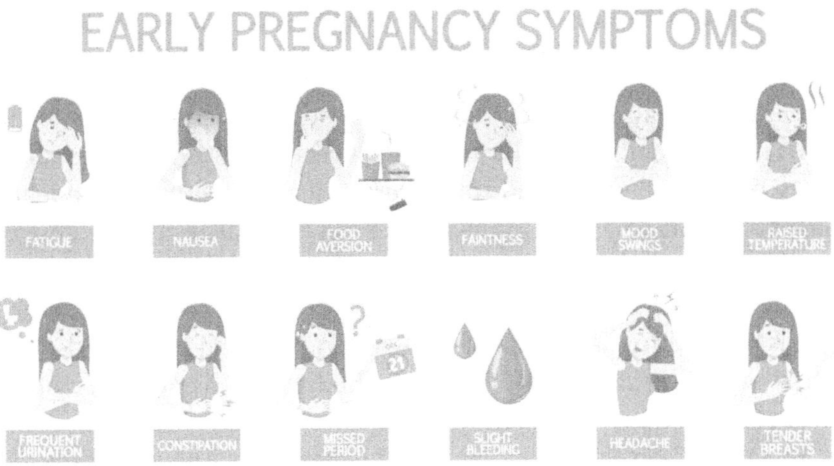

INTRODUCTION

It's never in every case, simply comprehending what's in store as a first-time mom. From the moment you find you're pregnant and share this with the individual nearest to you, most, as a rule, your significant other, accomplice or sperm contributor, your head unavoidably is by all accounts in a spiral. Mind you the disclosure itself may represent its very own arrangement of inquiries however we'll leave that for another theme of discourse. You understand that presently it's happened what's straightaway. You question the fate of your activity whenever utilized, your way of life, how it'll change your present circumstance, and it goes on. This much is valid, having an infant without a doubt changes the dynamic of everything in your life, and it does as such to improve things.

Whenever you ask yourself, when is the best time to tell your manager the 'uplifting news'? In case you're similar to a lot of ladies out there, you may have found you're pregnant. It's upsetting enough attempting to dazzle the questioner. However, the additional weight of realizing that you're four months pregnant, not indicating at this time and making a decent attempt to persuade the potential manager of your responsibility and accessibility to begin working with no predictable motivation to be off work anytime inside the following year is sufficient to make you cry, which you do following the meeting in the restroom slow down.

There is additionally the million-dollar question of when to come back to work. Your particular condition would direct what might be ideal. If a solitary parent, you may find that 'the sooner, the better' is the leading choice accessible to you, particularly on the off chance that you have no help whatsoever. As anyone might expect even wedded couples banter with one another on whether the principle workers compensation/pay can bolster a group of at least three while the spouse is off work during the first not many months. Children in the underlying stages or months don't request that a lot other than nappies, garments and reasonable travel when out on the town. The special reward is breastfeeding, as no cash should be spent on containers, sterilizers, and perhaps breast siphon. Mind you, and you do need to be guided on the most proficient method to hook the child on appropriately. To know that there is no milk in the first not many days, yet colostrum and that your areolas will get sore at some stage or other.

Even though not extremely reassuring in the first place, I guarantee you, it improves. What is most remunerating is seeing your little one being fed absolutely with your milk. The therapeutic ways of thinking exceptionally support the comfort of breastfeeding. They additionally support that the child is benefited from interest. In this manner, there is no requirement for the arrangement of any kind. The most you may require is open to a nursing bra and breast cushions, the rest you leave to your suckling little beloved newborn.

REACTIONS FOR THE PREGNANCY

How I found out ____

____

____

The first thing I did ____

____

____

My boyfriend's and friends' reactions ______________________

____

____

____

____

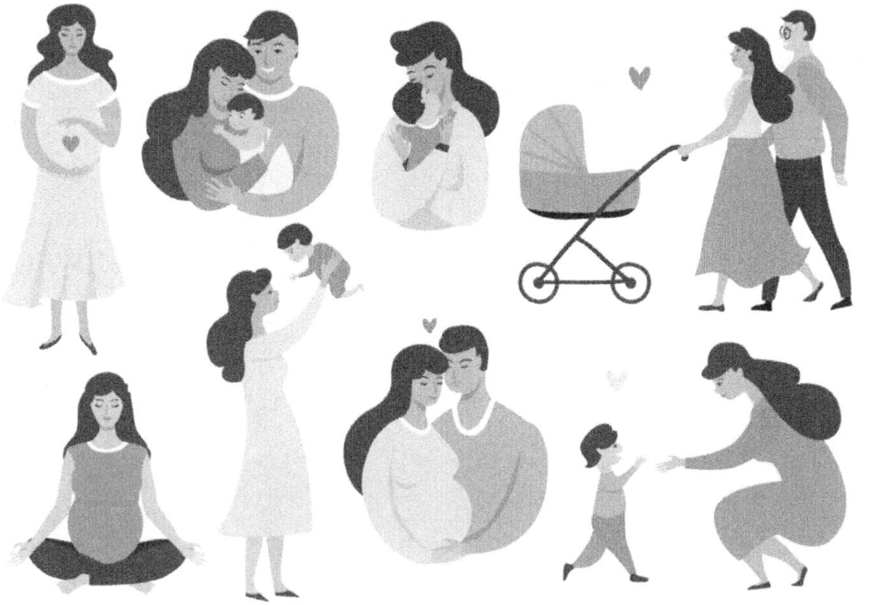

"A baby fills a place in your heart that you never knew was empty." - *Unknown*

CHAPTER ONE

FORMULA FOR A HEALTHY JOYOUS PREGNANCY

The Joy of Being a First Time Mom

You discover that you are pregnant and the entirety of the abrupt your whole world is turned upside off guard by the plan. On the off chance that you are in any way similar to me, you are terrified, excited, apprehensive, energized, restless and anxious. You have positively no clue what is going to happen to your body, your life, your home and your association with your accomplice. Trust me! As startling as everything may appear its merits, and every second your body is going to experience a considerable amount of changes. Your breasts will get enormous, firm and adjust. Your belly will seem as though you are conveying a watermelon. You may or not get stretch imprints. You will sweat, need to pee always, be worn out, eager and particular the subsequent you look at your beautiful infant the entirety of the hopelessness you suffered for nine months will blur away.

As a first-time pregnant lady, you will have a considerable amount of inquiries. Record them as you proceed to ask your Phencyclidine (PCP) at your visits. You may imagine that a portion of your questions is senseless, yet it is your PCP's business to answer them and assist you with feeling quiet during the procedure. Try not to spare a moment to call the specialist or medical caretaker if you figure something is not right. It is smarter to be sheltered than sorry. You can likewise go to your sweethearts for answers, proposals and tips during your pregnancy, labour and first year of parenthood.

Having a child can be one of the most extraordinary encounters. Here are a few hints for a first-time Mom to assist you with overcoming the harsher times. Most ladies today, are working when they become pregnant. That implies settling on a choice whether to remain at home with the child or come back to work. This is something you can consider during your pregnancy, gauging the advantages and disadvantages of your salary, versus the benefits to this kid, and any others to come later on. If you choose to go back to work, discovering childcare early will alleviate you of the stresses when your maternity leave is at an end.

Ladies who work all day, regularly wind up overwhelmed in things that identify with the child, regardless of whether it's their clothing, their rest plans, or their feedings. Now and again it can appear as though your entire life rotates around them, where it is used to include associates, companions and visits to family. One of the essential hints for a first-time Mom is that you shouldn't surrender as long as you can remember to the enhanced one that you're conveying. After the infant is conceived, you will be their essential guardian. However, you shouldn't be attached to them consistently. Set aside a few minutes for you, regardless of whether it's a yoga class around evening time with Dad doing the looking after children, a date out with your accomplice, and one of the grandparents ruining the new debut.

Significantly, you have a break from the steady focal point of your ordinary exercises with the child. This can incorporate numerous at-home practices. Also, such as perusing, stitching, or even artworks that you delighted in before the birth. The child will be similarly as cheerful watching you lose and engaged with your side interest, as they would be if you were doing the clothing. You may even discover a gathering for moms at your congregation or nearby public venue. Sharing tips for a first-time Mom with others is one method for facilitating the weights and stress of whether you are doing things right, and the time out, even with an infant, will be an adjustment in the schedule that you'll greet!

Challenges and Possible Solutions For First Time Mom

It is relatively overwhelming to be a first-time mother, regardless of how old she is. Likewise, it is difficult for her to envision what it resembles to be a first-time mom, irrespective of the amount she attempts to set herself up already. The following are a portion of my encounters a woman had when she had her first child and a few arrangements that have overcome those challenges.

1. Lack of certainty: I recall when I had my first infant; I didn't have a clue how to hold her. The attendant in the emergency

clinic just passed the child to me despondently because I demanded breast nourishing her. At the point when she saw that I was holding the infant mistakenly, she condemned me, saying that I would break the child's neck. I felt so embarrassed about myself. I had gone for pre-birth classes, and I knew the hypothesis of how to hold an infant, yet with regards to the viable part, I had no clue how I should convey the infant. The arrangement: Be certain and realize that you have in-conceived mother nature. Try not to let either the medical caretakers or specialists drive you around. On the off chance that you are uncertain of anything, ask first. Get your better half to remain with you for some time.

2. Postnatal wretchedness: After I returned from the medical clinic after delivery, I went into the gloom. I was feeling extremely lousy. I thought that the entire world was against me. I felt so pathetic. The most exceedingly terrible part was that my better half couldn't comprehend why I was discouraged. He couldn't see the motivation behind why I ought to be discouraged. That time, we didn't have the foggiest idea about that most ladies experience postnatal sorrow after delivery. Along these lines, he felt that I was troublesome, and I continued crying and crying. I was worried and baffled always. We were unquestionably not set up for this. The arrangement: Be set up for postnatal discouragement, talk about it before the delivery. Certain teas would help with the downturn when you know about it, you would be all the more tolerating of the circumstance and will receive in return quicker. You can likewise apply some sweet-smelling oil, for example, jasmine oil to lessen the misery. All the more

critically, consistently get enough rest.

3. Challenges with family members. Among all these bedlams of changing with my new job as a mother, there were likewise issues with over-minding family members who came to visit. They rushed to pass judgment, yet delayed to comprehend. They couldn't stand by to play with the infant and didn't care for the child to rest when they are wakeful. They demanded that everything ought to be done their direction. There were additionally a ton of 'good-natured' family members who gave a great deal of hypothesis, however little hands-on help. The arrangement: Again, you were given the infant, do what you believe is best for the infant. You will locate that even with consequent infants, there aren't finished "most popular strategies" to provide food for all. Each new child is another experience, and it is extraordinary. At the point when I had my third little girl, I imagined that I knew a great deal since I previously had two at the same time, she refuted me! In this way, you and your child will discover your harmony! Here are a few hints. It is great to get somebody near you to remain for some time, the first 2 to about a month - Attempt to get your significant other to stay at home also. While you needn't bother with a lot of family members pestering you, 1 or 2 can be useful during this period. Delay or maintain a strategic distance from any visits from benevolent family members. Instruct them to come half a month.

More or less, I feel that it is significant that a first-time mom has a care group that can assist her with experiencing the underlying time of being a mom. This should begin when she is pregnant. It has a great deal of effect when she realizes that there are many individuals out there that are experiencing or have experienced what she is also passing through, that she isn't the only one that she isn't the one in particular that is confronting this challenge.

Step by step instructions to Treat Stress During Pregnancy

Pregnancy is an excellent and glad time; however, it can likewise be loaded up with uncertainty and uneasiness. Various conditions can prompt worry during your pregnancy, including fluctuating hormone levels, vulnerability about the future, physical distress, or a previous mental issue. On the off chance that you are focused on, you may encounter trouble sleeping, cerebral pains, hustling heartbeat, and over the top musings. It is essential to recollect pressure doesn't just influence you. Research demonstrates that reliable high-tension levels may affect the advancement of your child. In any case, there are various approaches to treat pressure.

Research demonstrates that steady high uneasiness levels may influence the improvement of your infant. Be that as it may, there are various approaches to treat pressure usually, without depending on anxiolytics.

Instructions to Treat Stress Naturally During Pregnancy

• Find your triggers — Is there anything explicit that makes you on edge? Focus on what's going on when you feel generally worried.

• Get Some Rest — Exhaustion or unpredictable sleeping propensities can prompt expanded negative feelings, including pressure. Be sure that you are permitting yourself a lot of rest.

• Eat vigorously — A well-adjusted diet can help diminish worry, just as keeping you and your infant reliable.

• Exercise — Thirty minutes of gentle to direct practice a few days seven days is gigantically advantageous. It can likewise help lower cortisol levels, which is the hormone that causes uneasiness.

• Meditation — Meditating can help clear your brain and lower your feelings of anxiety.

• Therapy — If your feelings of anxiety become excruciating, you might need to look for an advisor, to examine conceivable hidden issues underneath your nervousness, just as reliable approaches to adapt to your sentiments.

Step by step instructions to Treat Stress when Naturally Doesn't Work

On the off chance that you have pursued the above advances regardless you feel continually on edge, you may need to converse with your medicinal services supplier about potentially beginning anxiolytics. There are various. Various prescriptions are sheltered to take while you are pregnant. Stress is essential during pregnancy, and there is nothing amiss with looking for treatment, in the manner in which works best for you.

Pregnancy Emotions

Changing feelings are, for some ladies, one of the most widely recognized reactions during pregnancy. It tends to be disappointing and debilitating to move to start with one feeling then onto the next and be not able to clarify what emotion you are feeling and why. For the individuals who were not enthusiastic preceding pregnancy, this invasion of pregnancy feelings might be particularly surprising.

Reasons for Pregnancy Emotions

First, it's essential to remind yourself not to feel regretful or embarrassed, on the off chance that you are in a specific enthusiastic state. Uplifted pregnancy feelings are not out of the ordinary. There are numerous outside and inside variables which can cause an expansion in your passionate country during pregnancy, and it doesn't mean you are "moody" or "crazy." Pregnancy feelings are an ordinary piece of advancement.

Hormones

During pregnancy, ladies experience an expansion in the generation of hormones, for example, progesterone and estrogen, contingent upon how far along they are in their pregnancy. This increment in hormones can affect your feelings and your mind's capacity to screen those feelings. This is exceptionally normal and ought not to be a reason for concern except if you wind up in a condition of severe enthusiastic unsteadiness and trouble.

Stress

For some reasons, pregnancy can expedite extra pressure. While beginning, a family is energizing and loaded up with a great deal of euphoria, as the pregnancy advances you might be worried about the progressions it will bring. Pregnant ladies may wind up concerned about the future, funds, lodging, backing, work, and medicinal consideration. This pressure can make feelings arise, and occupy from self-care that may assist better with dealing with these feelings.

Body Changes and Body Image

A few ladies may encounter more physical distress during their pregnancy than others. As the body changes for your developing infant, you may face numerous physical inconveniences, from morning disorder to body throbs. Body picture issues may make you feel less physically alluring, as you look in the mirror and see a portion of the adjustments in your body. Any of these things can affect both mental and physical wellbeing, which adds to pressure and can cause an interruption in ordinary feelings.

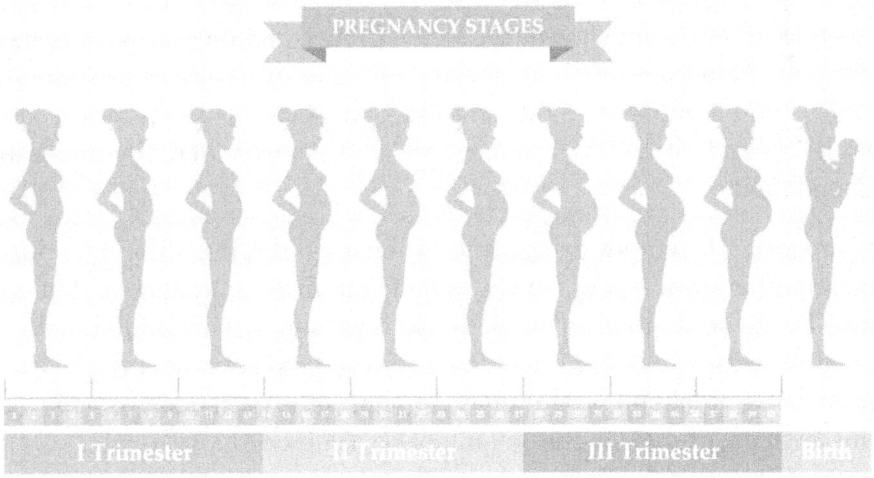

Weariness

Regardless of whether from inconvenience or stress, numerous ladies may encounter trouble sleeping during pregnancy. Absence of rest has been appeared to affect an individual's enthusiastic state profoundly. Along these lines, if your pregnancy is causing transparent dreams or making rest troublesome, this can propagate an elevated excited state and make feelings hard to oversee.

Approaches to Cope with Pregnancy Emotions

While it might appear to be overpowering, there are numerous things you can do to adapt and make your feelings increasingly reasonable.

A few recommendations include:

• Self-care: Listen to your body and mind and know about what you need. On the off chance that an air pocket shower sounds unwinding, do it. On the off chance that you need time alone to relax and peruse a book or get a pedicure, set aside a few minutes for it.

• Sleep: Getting 8 hours of good rest can do astonishing things for your enthusiastic state. While this may not generally be conceivable, do all that you can to get a reliable measure of rest. You can try different things with sleeping positions, let your accomplice know whether you are experiencing issues sleeping so you two can think of an arrangement to ensure you are getting the rest you need.

• Diet: Like rest, what you eat is an incredibly common approach to help with your mood and feelings. Eating well and everyday nourishments, rather than prepared food sources, advances both physical and psychological wellness, which adds to expanded enthusiastic dependability.

• Support: A empowering and robust gathering of individuals encompassing you is fantastically significant during pregnancy. Making close loved ones mindful of your feelings and having individuals to converse with when you feel overpowered is very useful for your enthusiastic wellbeing. Sometimes, if you are experiencing issues with your feelings, proficient guiding might be a choice to investigate.

Pregnancy can be a lovely time, yet it's imperative to be set up for the progressions that may happen in your enthusiastic state. It is critical to recollect pregnancy feelings are typical and not to feel regretful for the variety of emotions you are feeling yet to know about them and react reliably and positively.

Inform your primary care physician as to whether you have a feeling that your feelings are amazingly temperamental, you are encountering severe misery, or having considerations of suicide. In these cases, therapeutic intercession or expert guiding might be fundamental.

MY FIRST FEELINGS AND THOUGHTS

Negative sides ______________________

____

____

____

Positive sides ______________________

____

____

____

____

My boyfriend's opinion ______________________________

____

____

Vote for myself: __________ Vote for my boyfriend: __________

Exercise Guidelines for Pregnancy

On the off chance that you have been following a regular exercise program before your pregnancy, you ought to have the option to keep up that program somewhat all through your pregnancy. Exercise doesn't expand the danger of premature delivery in a healthy, generally safe pregnancy. The significant thing is to talk about these pregnancy exercise rules with your medicinal services supplier and set up the correct daily schedule for you.

Rules

• If you are beginning an exercise program as a method for improving your wellbeing during your pregnancy, you should start gradually and be mindful so as not to overexert yourself. Consider a pre-birth yoga class that is explicitly intended for pregnant ladies.

• Listen to your body. Your body will typically give you flag that the time has come to decrease the degree of exercise you are performing.

• Never exercise to the point of weariness or shortness of breath. This is an indication that your child and your body can't get the oxygen they need.

• Wear agreeable exercise footwear that gives a stable lower leg and curves support.

- Take visit breaks, and drink a lot of liquids during exercise.
- Avoid practicing in incredibly blistering climate.
- Avoid rough territory or dangerous ground when running or cycling. Your joints are laxer in pregnancy, so lower leg sprains and different wounds may happen.
- Contact sports ought to be abstained from during pregnancy.
- Weight preparing ought to underscore improving tone, particularly in the chest area and stomach region. Abstain from lifting loads over your head and utilizing loads that strain the lower back muscles.
- During the second and third trimesters, maintain a strategic distance from exercise that includes lying level on your back as this reduction's bloodstream to the uterus.
- Include unwinding and extending when your exercise program.
- Eat a sound diet that incorporates a lot of natural products, vegetables, and complex sugars.

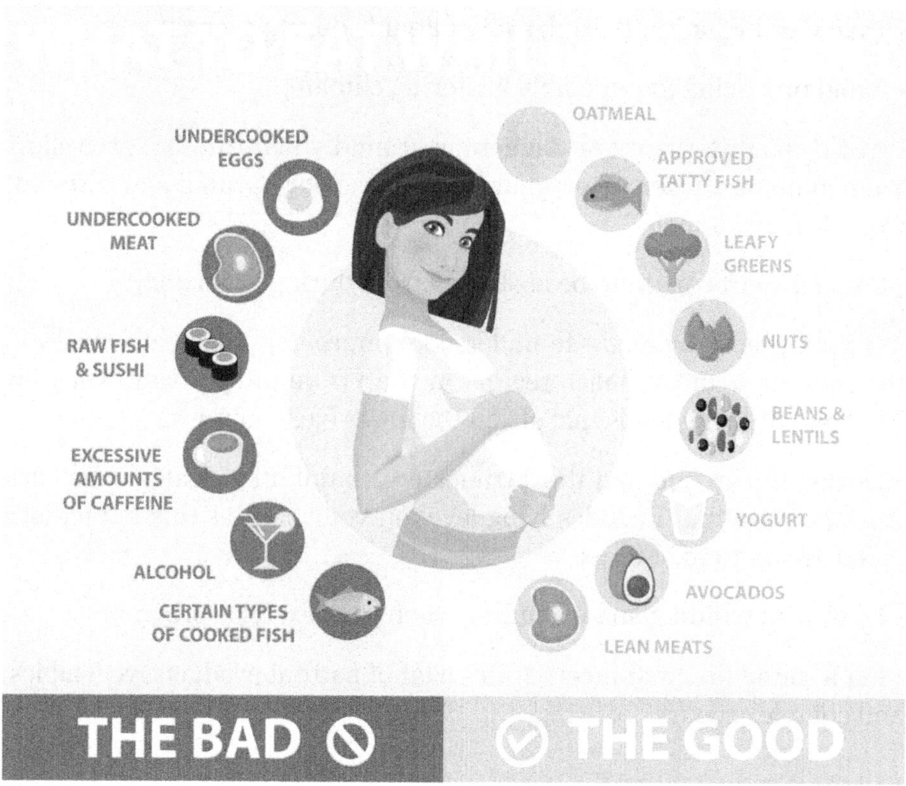

Pregnancy Nutrition

A nutritious, well-adjusted eating plan can be perhaps the best blessing you provide for your creating infant. Pregnancy nutrition is fundamental to a stable infant. Preferably, embracing a right dieting arrangement before pregnancy is ideal. Regardless of how long are left on your commencement schedule, it's never past the point where it is possible to begin! Providing your own body with a delicious mix of nutritious nourishments can improve your richness, keep you feeling sound during pregnancy, and make ready for more uncomplicated labour.

It can likewise set up central structure squares of development and by and significant wellbeing for your kid. The nourishment we eat regularly influences how our bodies work, how we recuperate and develop, and how we keep up vitality and quality for quite a long time to come. It additionally decides the fundamental nutritional wellbeing that our youngsters are brought into the world and gives a model to their dietary patterns during adolescence and past.

Pregnancy is the one time in your life when your dietary patterns legitimately influence someone else. Your choice to fuse tasty vegetables, entire grains and vegetables, lean protein, and generally nourishment decisions into your eating plan previously and during pregnancy will give your child a trustworthy beginning throughout everyday life.

Pregnancy Nutrition: Weight Change and Calories

Your body will put on weight during your pregnancy! As you watch your weight start to expand, accept it as verification that your body is sustaining your developing child. When you are prepared to conceive an offspring, your complete blood volume will have expanded by as much as 60%. Your breasts will have loaded up with milk. Your uterus will have developed to suit your child and has loaded up with amniotic liquid. Your child has grown to gauge 6 to 10 pounds (by and large). To achieve these gainful changes, your body needs around 300 additional calories for each day during your second and third trimester of pregnancy.

Each lady ought to examine her individual nutritional needs with her social insurance supplier. Try not to disregard your child's wellbeing by ignoring your own!

Fantasy: Now that you are pregnant, you ought to eat for two.

Truth: without a doubt, your supplement needs increment, yet vitality prerequisites increment by around 300 calories for each day for the second and third trimester of pregnancy.

Fantasy: Gaining less weight during pregnancy will make delivery simpler.

Actuality: Mothers who don't put on enough weight during pregnancy place their infants in danger for extreme complexities, for example, untimely birth, which can cause lung and heart issues.

Fantasy: If you put on the perfect measure of weight during pregnancy, none of it will be fat increase.

Actuality: A healthy pregnancy incorporates fat stockpiling. Your body utilizes this overabundance fat as vitality during labour and breastfeeding.

Fantasy: Pregnant ladies ache for the nourishment their bodies need.

Reality: Pregnant ladies can long for nourishments of any kind. Desires ought not to be the sole marker of nutritional needs.

Fantasy: A pregnant lady who is solid won't encounter distresses.

Reality: Nausea, acid reflux, and obstruction are not one-sided! They will beset ladies paying little mind to sound living. Be that as it may, ladies who usually eat well nourishments, drink a lot of water, exercise consistently, and keep away from abundance sugar and fat may fundamentally lessen these awkward manifestations.

Pregnancy Nutrition: Food Groups

It is useful to focus on the prescribed everyday servings from every nutrition type. Most nourishments accompany a nutrition name connected. This nutrition mark will assist you in knowing what sum comprises one meal.

Protein

Specialists prescribe 75 to 100 grams of protein for each day. Protein decidedly influences the development of fetal tissue, including the cerebrum. It likewise helps your breast and uterine tissue to develop during pregnancy, and it assumes a job in your expanding blood supply.

Instances of every day wellsprings of protein:

2-3 servings of meat (1 serving = roughly 3 ounces/size of a deck of cards)

• Fully cooked fish or fish

• Liver

• Chicken

• Lean meat

• Lamb

• Pork

• Nuts (1 serving = roughly ⅓ cup)

• Tofu (1 serving = roughly ½ cup)

2-3 servings of vegetables (1 serving = roughly ½ cup)

• Split peas

• Red and white kidney beans

• Black beans

• Navy beans

• Black-looked at peas

• Chickpeas (garbanzo beans)

Calcium

The everyday necessity of calcium is around 1000 milligrams during pregnancy. Calcium enables your body to direct liquids, and it helps manufacture your infant's bones and tooth buds.

Instances of day by day wellsprings of calcium:

3-4 servings of dairy

• Milk (1 serving = 1 cup)

• Eggs (1 serving = 1 enormous egg)

• Yogurt (1 serving = 1 cup)

• Pasteurized cheddar (1 serving = around 1.5 ounces or four playing dice stacked together)

• Tofu (1 serving = ½ cup)

• White beans (1 serving = around ½ cup)

• Almonds (1 serving = around ⅓ cup)

• Salmon (1 serving = around 3 ounces)

• Turnip greens (1 serving = around 1 cup)

• Cabbage (1 serving = around 1 cup)

Iron

In blend with sodium, potassium, and water, iron helps increment your blood volume and anticipates frailty. A day by day admission of 27 milligrams is perfect during pregnancy.

Instances of day by day wellsprings of iron:

2-3 servings of verdant green vegetables (1 serving = around 1 cup)

- Collard
- Turnip
- Spinach
- Lettuce
- Cabbage

Three servings of entire grains (1 serving = around ½ cup or one cut)

- Bread
- Cornmeal
- Cereal
- Oatmeal

2-3 servings of lean protein (1 serving = around 3 ounces/size of a deck of cards)

- Beef
- Seafood
- Poultry

Folate/Folic Acid

Folic corrosive assumes a vital job in decreasing the danger of neural cylinder absconds, including spina bifida. Specialists prescribe 600 to 800 micrograms (.6 to .8 milligrams) every day.

Instances of every day wellsprings of folate:

Two servings of dull green verdant vegetables (1 serving = around 1 cup)

- Collard

- Turnip
- Spinach
- Lettuce
- Cabbage

2-3 servings of the natural product (1 serving = around ½ cup)

- Orange
- Strawberry
- Lemon
- Mango
- Tomato
- Grapefruit
- Kiwi
- Melon

Three serving of entire grain (1 serving = roughly ½ cup or one cut)

- Bread
- Cornmeal
- Cereal
- Oatmeal

Two servings of vegetables (1 serving = roughly ½ cup)

- Split peas
- Red and white kidney beans
- Black beans
- Navy beans
- Black-looked at peas
- Chickpeas (garbanzo beans)

PERSONAL OR RECOMMENDED RECIPES

Name:

Ingredients	Instructions
▪	
▪	
▪	
▪	
▪	

Name:

Ingredients	Instructions
▪	
▪	
▪	
▪	
▪	

Name:

Ingredients	Instructions
▪	
▪	
▪	
▪	

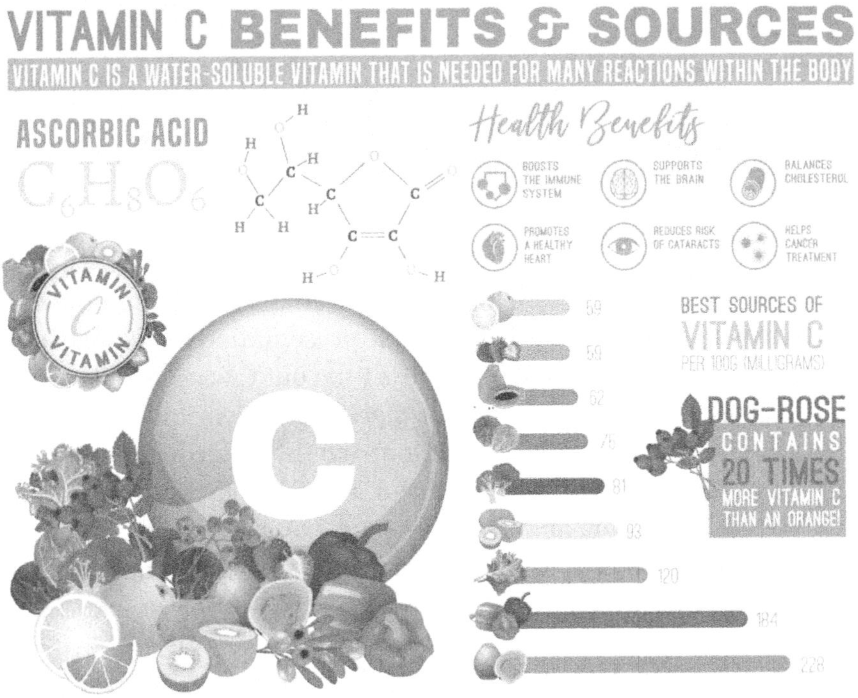

VITAMIN C BENEFITS & SOURCES
VITAMIN C IS A WATER-SOLUBLE VITAMIN THAT IS NEEDED FOR MANY REACTIONS WITHIN THE BODY
ASCORBIC ACID
Health Benefits
BOOSTS THE IMMUNE SYSTEM
SUPPORTS THE BRAIN
BALANCES CHOLESTEROL
PROMOTES A HEALTHY HEART
REDUCES RISK OF CATARACTS
HELPS CANCER TREATMENT
BEST SOURCES OF VITAMIN C
PER 100G (MILLIGRAMS)
DOG-ROSE CONTAINS 20 TIMES MORE VITAMIN C THAN AN ORANGE!
59
59
62
76
81
93
120
184
228

Nutrient C

Products of the soil plentiful in Vitamin C will advance injury mending, tooth and bone improvement, and metabolic procedures. Specialists prescribe at any rate 85 milligrams for every day.

Instances of every day wellsprings of Vitamin C:

Three servings of natural product or vegetables (1 serving = around ½ cup)

- Orange
- Strawberry
- Lemon
- Mango
- Tomato
- Grapefruit

• Kiwi

• Melon

• Potato

• Peppers

Other Nutritional Concerns

During pregnancy, a few nourishments can make hurt a creating child. Be sure that all meats are cooked to evade presentation to toxoplasmosis, salmonella, and other unsafe microbes. Take out tobacco smoke, sedate use, and liquor utilization from your diet. Decrease or take out charged refreshments (pop, espresso) from your day by day consumption, and keep up a sensible exercise program all through your pregnancy. Strolling and swimming are viewed as solid exercises during pregnancy; however, consistently counsel with your social insurance supplier before beginning another exercise program.

Keeping Yourself Happy During Pregnancy

Pregnancy is the first period in a lady's life. When you're pregnant, you are loaded with satisfaction, trust and uneasiness. Individuals give you favours, advice and that additional consideration that makes you feel exceptional. Keeping yourself cheerful during all the three trimesters is entirely up to you. It is essential to be bright and feel happy while pregnant, as your passionate prosperity legitimately influences infant's neurological and mental advancement. Studies have demonstrated that increasingly glad pregnant ladies are, the more they are probably going to convey a sound child.

Yet, how to be glad during pregnancy? We comprehend that the circumstance around each pregnant lady is extraordinary, and they need not generally be happy ones always. In any case, you need to try to channel your attitude for being glad during pregnancy.

Bliss consistently exists in yourself. As you gear up for the approaching labour, each trimester will introduce different sorts of circumstances for you to manage. From that irritating morning infection to excruciating mood swings, you will have a bunch of petty challenges to manage. The following are some specific shot ways on the most proficient method to remain glad during pregnancy that can assist you with staying in front of different issues and be unequivocally cheerful:

1. Act naturally:

Pregnancy is uncommon. Regardless of how hindered you are with various musings; it is essential to 'be'.

- Being in the circumstance and concentrating on your infant causes you to handle different issues all the more adequately.

- As the most significant thing for you would be your infant, everything will look worth battling for.

- Being inherently glad while tending to littler issues falls into place without a hitch once you are yourself.

2. Keep up A Healthy Lifestyle:

Way of life influences how you are and the method in which you work in regular day to day existence.

- A dynamic way of life which is sound and beneficial consistently accomplishes all the more magnificent.

- Once you are pregnant, there is each opportunity that awkwardness would set in.

- You would begin feeling more dormant and sluggish than previously.

- Making a conscious endeavour to pursue positive routine affects your intuition as it were.

- The more you eat right and remain fit, the more you will begin creating sound and upbeat musings.

- A stable life clears a path for a sound personality!

3. Avoid Negative People:

A few people and circumstances are regularly alluded to as 'dangerous' in light of how they make you feel.

• Hanging around with individuals who are doubters and getting by in a situation that is loaded down with misery is an enormous calamity on the off chance that you are pregnant.

• Stay away from adverse words, musings and activities, and above all, individuals who show them.

• This is no time to enjoy additional pressure and cause weight to your brain and heart.

4. Yoga And Meditation:

For quite a long time, yoga and reflection have demonstrated to be a shelter to pregnant ladies.

• Undergo a decent yoga session with a prepared proficient.

• You will start to feel revived, solid and glad.

• The breathing exercises are said to discharge the enthusiastic poisons and modify your reasoning example.

• Try to go through, at any rate, 30 minutes consistently doing yoga and contemplation. You will locate a significant contrast in the manner you feel.

5. Keep up A Journal:

It is energizing to record how you feel and what you experience during pregnancy.

• These recollections recorded in content and video structures proceed to become lifetime recollections.

• Spend additional time recording the first encounters; the first kick, the first compression, the first child shower, and so on.

• Shoot recordings that intrigue you.

• You might need to flaunt every one of these diaries to your youngster years after their appearance.

6. Treat Others Kindly:

Treating others benevolently may now and again become touchy, on account of the repulsive mood swings that negatively affect your passionate parity.

• You will be effectively angered and passionate during barely any stages while you are pregnant.

• Understand this isn't your issue.

• At a similar time, don't show your aggravated side to everyone around you.

• Try and control your irregular motivations. It might be hard to do as such, however treating others severely will likewise wind up making you feel remorseful and troubled.

7. Appreciate All That Preparation:

Before the appearance of your child, you will be occupied with making arrangements.

• Right from orchestrating the nursery to looking for pregnancy and your infant, you will be brimming with enthusiasm as you plan and sort things.

• Enjoy the arrangements without limit.

• Relish each moment as you consume on your needs and that of your baby's.

8. Spoil Yourself:

This is the ideal time to rest every one of your stresses and enjoy.

• Make sure you keep arrangements of spa and body knead.

• Get that since a long time ago planned body conditioning and pedicure ceremonies.

• Once your child shows up, you won't be as fortunate with available time as you are currently.

• You will be astounded at the sort of joy and help that accompanies some magnificence treatment.

9. Representative Work:

Most times, pregnant ladies feel like they are solitary warriors set to assume control over the approaching obligation of parenthood.

• This sort of self-troubling is of no advantage, except stressing you both physically and inwardly.

• Feel allowed to request help and representative work to the individuals in your home.

• In case you are a single parent, recognize those select companions of yours who will come accommodating in times of emergency post-delivery.

• Delegating a touch of work to others will empower you to concentrate on investing more energy with your infant.

10. Relax:

Breathing profoundly surges in marvelous musings that outcome is similarly encouraging activities.

• The more you centre around your breath and settle down, the more loosened up you will be at the time of labour.

• What increasingly, breathing goes far in helping you dispose of negative contemplations and challenges like post birth anxiety.

• These essential hints are very successful in improving you with cheerful emotions and positive contemplations.

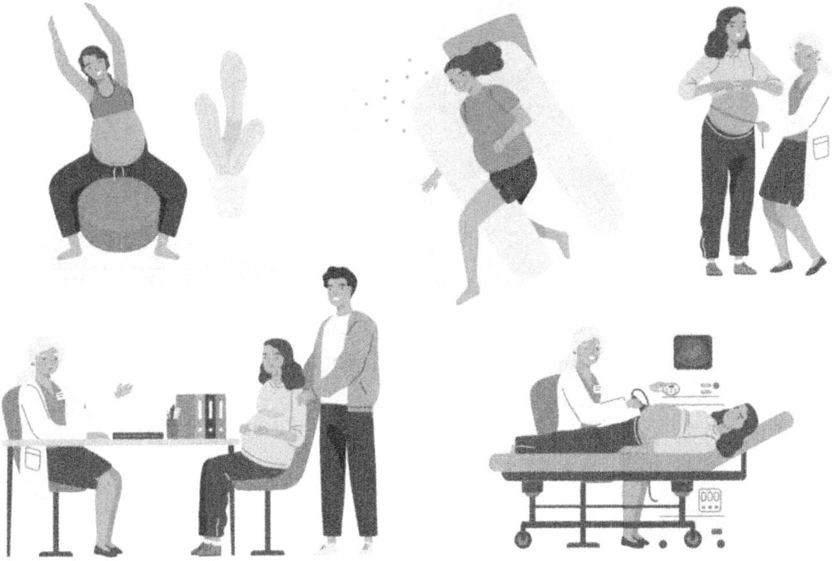

"The most important thing she'd learned over the years was that there was no way to be a perfect mother and a million ways to be a good one." – *Jill Churchill*

CHAPTER TWO

EVERYTHING TO EXPECT FROM EACH TRIMESTER

State the word 'pregnant', and you will have ladies of any age swooping down on you with expressions of guidance. The lethal disclaimer will uphold each announcement they articulate, "I talk as a matter of fact", and thus you will be in issue – to trust them or not?

Pregnancy Myths

While some of them have been precluded totally, there are still a few myths that have been doing the rounds for such a large number of decades that we have mostly come to acknowledge these as valid without endeavouring to find the genuine truth behind them. Here we present you the best 23 broadly accepted pregnancy myths and the real truth:

Myth 1: Belly Position Determines Baby's Gender:

The odds are that any forecast your aunt or relative or any local lady wills have a 50% plausibility of working out as expected. Consider it. It has nothing to do with belly positions. Every lady unexpectedly conveys her child, and everything relies on body type and hip estimations. The sex of the child unquestionably has nothing to do with it.

Myth 2: Certain Types of Foods Will Affect Baby's Complexion:

This one is ridiculous. Your precious ladies attempt to push you into drinking a lot of coconut water with the sound guidance that it will cause you to have a reasonable infant. Some old-timers even venture to such an extreme as to instruct you to remain off iron enhancements since they make your infant's skin dull. First of all, nourishment has nothing to do with appearance. Also, remaining off iron enhancements may prompt actual results both for the mother and the infant. Thus, this is one legend you ought to dismiss.

Myth 3: You Should Eat for Two:

Regardless of what anybody says, you don't have to eat for two. Indeed, pregnancy increases your day by day caloric prerequisite. However, just by 300 calories. This implies only a single chapatti with ghee, or two servings of natural product, or two servings of the plate of mixed greens extra. Not the sort of nourishment fleeting trend that is recommended to you since you have another life developing inside you.

Myth 4: Eating Spicy Foods Will Lead to Labor Induction:

No chance. Eating zesty will prompt indigestion and gases. Not labour acceptance as is advised to you time and once more. Be that as it may, to lessen uneasiness from gas inconvenience, which might be even painful for a pregnant lady in fragile wellbeing, it is fitting to devour zesty stuff in moderate amount.

Myth 5: More Heartburn Means More Hair on Baby's Scalp!

The measure of hair on an infant depends a great deal on the hereditary make-up of the youngster and not founded on how much acid reflux the mother endures during pregnancy. The developing load of the embryo frequently prompts pushing the stomach related mechanical assembly upwards towards the heart sphincter, prompting corrosive arrangement. This is the purpose behind hyperacidity and not hair. Ladies with fabulous acid refluxes have brought forth bare infants, and innumerable ladies with nay indigestion have had youngsters with substantial hairs on their heads.

Myth 6: No Sex during Pregnancy:

While most specialists may encourage you to remain off sex during the first three months, they all concur that during the second and third trimesters, it is basically protected. Additionally, numerous ladies experience an expansion in sexual want because of an increment in the hormone levels. Embryos are ensured by layers of tissues, and can't be hurt by intercourse. So except if your expert has explicitly instructed you to avoid sex if it's not too much trouble keep getting private with your accomplice.

Myth 7: Eclipses Can Cause Genetic Defects:

Congenital fissures and palates are hereditary abnormalities and are caused because of certain hereditary variables inclining to it. They are all the more regularly found in intermarriages. By no means are they identified with shrouds both of the sun or the moon?

Myth 8: Spinal Anesthesia Causes Backaches:

While spinal anesthesia may contribute to some degree to spinal pains, they are fundamentally brought about by the moving focus of gravity in pregnant ladies. Every one of that weight a hopeful mother conveys makes the spine bend unreasonably prompting ungainly situating and spinal pain. Indeed, even ladies who usually carry experience the ill effects of incapacitating spinal illnesses, and the best way to anticipate it is by doing spine-fortifying exercises both during and after pregnancy.

Myth 9: Ghee for Easy Labor and Delivery:

Benevolent aunts will guide you to expend ghee in overflowing sums, probably because ghee greases up the birth channel, in this way encouraging simple labour and delivery. This specific legend has no base at all and having ghee in high amount will make you put on over the top measure of weight! The seriousness and span of labour contracts with each lady, and devouring ghee won't ease it in at any rate. Castor oil is regularly recommended by experts if work is postponed, to expedite the constrictions. However, ghee is only an old spouses' story.

Myth 10: Papaya Causes Abortion:

The premise behind this legend is that unripe or even semi-mature papaya contains latex that can enact uterine constrictions. Nonetheless, to cause unnatural birth cycle, a lady would need to expend papayas in humongous amount. Irregular birth cycles frequently happen due to inconsistencies in a hatchling, making it unviable for proceeding. You can undoubtedly make the most of your preferred products of the soil; however, much you might want, yet before that consistently affirm your diet with your primary care physician.

Myth 11: Determining The Sex Of The Baby, According To The Sexual Position:

Numerous ladies may have known about the 'thought' that the sex of the infant can be dictated by the sexual position embraced. In all actuality, you can't decide the child's sex by sexual situations, as they do not affect determining the sex of your infant.

Myth 12: Carrying Low Or High May Imply The Sex Of The Baby:

This is one of the most widely recognized myths related with pregnancy- during this period, the lady's body experiences a ton of changes relying upon the situation of the hatchling, muscle size and the fat kept around her stomach area that shows the size and state of a pregnant lady. There is no probability of conveying high is a young lady and carrying low is a kid, which is a typical legend discovered circling among numerous ladies.

Myth 13: Morning Sickness Can Determine The Sex Of Your Baby:

Morning ailment doesn't decide the infant's sex. Primarily, morning disorder happens because of a condition known as hyperemesis gravidarum. This condition is related with a sentiment of 'infection' as a rule on a vacant stomach or after the admission of specific prescriptions without the utilization of nourishment. Morning disorder is not the slightest bit identified with the sex of the infant.

Myth 14: Your Skin Becomes Dull During The Time Of Growth Of Your Baby:

It is a fantasy that is making rounds for a few ages now that when a ladies' skin gets dull during pregnancy, it is a direct result of the child's development. This isn't valid. Your body experiences changes as the bloodstream increment in every one of the cells. Numerous ladies experience sparkling skin, famously known as 'infant shine' and some may not work because of the idea of their body and irregular hormonal characteristics. In any case, there is no logical certainty supporting why a portion of the ladies don't get the 'child sparkle'. Rather than focusing on bluntness and sparkle, ladies ought to be mindful in keeping up a healthy diet with legitimate exercises, to improve their body quality.

Myth 15: Don't Sleep On Your Back:

During pregnancy, sleeping on your back may hinder blood dissemination in the body of your child. However, to date, there is no logical proof to help the way that sleeping on the back could be hurtful. The solace and uneasiness factors contrast from lady to lady. Sleeping on your left side is fitting as it builds the bloodstream to your lower body and back to the heart.

Myth 16: Avoid Raising Arms Above The Head While Pregnant:

This is one more legend – it is accepted that the umbilical rope may get folded over child's neck on the off chance that you raise your arms over your head during your pregnancy period. In any case, there is no proof to help the way that raising your arms could make the string get folded over your child. So don't hesitate to extend, play out the sun greeting and hold tight wet clothing as well.

Myth 17: Pregnant Women Shouldn't Bathe:

This may sound particularly entertaining, however honestly, there are myths like these creations adjust since a long while. During pregnancy, given the hormonal changes occurring, washing is significantly more significant than different times. Cleaning up doesn't hurt the child or the mother in any capacity. Be that as it may, care ought to be brought to chop down any potential dangers ensure that your shower water isn't excessively hot since the rise in temperature may cause specific issues.

Myth 18: Stress Is Bad For Fetus:

The vast majority of us accept that taking any worry during pregnancy is terrible for the embryo. In any case, late research shows that taking the moderate pressure is useful for the fetus. It quickens the advancement of the child and tones up the hatchling sensory system. Newborn children of moms who encountered a moderate degree of stress have quicker working cerebrums than moms without fear. Likewise, babies have higher mental and engine abilities destined to pressure experienced moms.

Myth 19: You Should Not Eat Sweets:

Chocolate is a particular major case. Studies uncover that pregnant ladies who have chocolate routinely will have babies who snicker all the more regularly and show less dread and grin. Likewise, pregnant ladies who will eat chocolate five and more times in seven days during the third trimester have 40% less danger of encountering hypertension.

Myth 20: You Should Stay Away From Seafood:

Another bogus proclamation. Eating bunches of fish high in omega-3 gives you more brilliant children. As per an examination, kids whose moms had at any rate 12 ounces of fish seven days had higher IQ, relational abilities, social and predominant engine aptitudes.

Myth 21: Expectant Mothers Feel Happy When Pregnant:

Indeed, it isn't valid. Pregnant ladies experience the ill effects of mood swings like some other ladies. About 20% of pregnant ladies will encounter tension and misery. Falling under despondency during pregnancy will build the odds of untimely conveyances or low birth weight.

Myth 22: You Should Stay Away From Your Pet:

It isn't valid. In any case, you ought not to change your pet's litter box as it can cause the danger of toxoplasmosis contamination. You can be that as it may snuggle your pet and it costs nothing.

Myth 23: Flying Will Increase Complications:

Not True. It is bogus once more. You may stress over the air terminal body scanners, X-beam machines and radiations from flying can influence your pregnancy. However, the sort of emissions won't enter much into the body. In this way, subsequently, they are probably not going to change the baby. Be that as it may, it isn't prudent to fly during the third trimester because there are chances you may convey on the way.

Most first time moms will in general fall prey to these senseless myths and might make endeavours to handle them, which may be dangerous for the child. You are most likely eased in the wake of looking at these pregnancy legend busters, yet at the same time, a good old aunt may demand to suffocate you in more myths. While you may go over these myths regularly, take all the competent natured counsel with a touch of salt and tune in to your therapeutic specialist.

What To Do And What Not To Do When Pregnant

Pregnancy acquires numerous physiological and mental changes in a lady. Also, you should be cautious about activities and not do. You should be set up for certain unanticipated conditions, yet try to realize how to keep yourself free from some undesirable stresses. On the off chance that you are pregnant and are anxious to think about things to incorporate and abstain from during the nine months.

MY FIRST CRAVING AND FOOLISHNESS

Craving ______________________________

____

____

____

Foolishness ______________________________

____

____

____

How dit it end? ______________________________

____

Things To Avoid During Pregnancy

There are numerous things you can't do while pregnant, for your infant's security and your wellbeing.

1. Do not eat raw meat, unpasteurized dairy, crude nourishments, singed food sources, and so forth. They may contain destructive organisms that can antagonistically influence you and your child's wellbeing. Such nourishments additionally add to unreasonable weight gain. At the point when you are eating crude foods grown from the ground, ensure that you are washing them thoroughly.

2. Do not paint the nursery as the synthetic compounds and solvents in the paints can be poisonous and hurtful. On the off chance that you need to decorate the nursery, at that point you can utilize normal or natural hues, and guarantee the room is well-ventilated.

3. Do not go over the edge on caffeine. It can build circulatory strain, pulse, and you need to go habitually to the loo. Likewise, caffeine goes through the placenta to the hatchling. It is additionally connected with an expanded danger of low birth weight and birth deserts.

4. Do not take meds without counselling your wellbeing professional. Certain meds may have specific measurement and ought not to be assumed control over-the-counter.

5. Do not wear stilettos and incline toward heels that are three-inch or less, for example, wedges, stages, and cat heels. Heels may make you awkward as the body's focal point of gravity changes and could subsequently bring about muscle harm, spinal pain, pelvic pain and loss of equalization. On the off chance that you have swollen lower legs, you may feel better in flip-flops.

6. Do not change the cat litter as the excrement can convey an uncommon parasitic illness, toxoplasmosis. Regardless of whether you do, wear gloves while changing and wash your hands after that.

7. Do not inhale smoke. It is connected to numerous intricacies including diseases, unexpected labour, unnatural birth cycle, low birth weight babies, abrupt newborn child demise disorder, and learning or conduct issues as the infant develops.

8. Do not take liquor, including wine, alcohol, and brew. It can go through the placenta and umbilical rope and influence the infant's creating mind and organs. Ordinary utilization of liquor may prompt untimely birth, cerebrum harm, unnatural birth cycle, stillbirth, and a deep-rooted crippling condition known as fetal liquor disorder.

9. Do not sit or represent expanded periods similarly situated. It can hurt the lower legs and veins. Take visit breaks and move around to keep your legs raised on the off chance that you have been on your feet for quite a while.

10. Do not become overly enthusiastic by conflicting data given in books, magazines, and online media. Trust your senses and if all else fails, converse with your expert.

11. Do not ingest illicit medications. Medications are related with expanded odds of low birth weight babies, weakened neurobehavioral improvement in babies, birth deformities, and withdrawal impacts.

12. Do not eat nourishments made of unpasteurized dairy items or uncooked/semi-cooked meat as they conceivably convey harmful microscopic organisms' listeria that makes you and your child defenceless against numerous sicknesses.

13. Do not get in contact with reptiles, for example, lizards, turtles, iguanas, and snakes. Their dung passes salmonella infection into your framework and can be perilous.

14. Ensure there are no ticks as their nibbles can cause Lyme sickness. The impacts remember lasting tooth staining for pregnant ladies and distortion of bones in the hatchling.

15. Avoid enhancements except if prompted by your medicinal services expert. Having unreasonable nutrient can inspire birth deserts in the child.

16. Stay away from video show terminals (VDTs), radios, high voltage electrical cables, transmit transmissions, and different other primary machines and correspondence gear. These produce hurtful, non-ionizing radiations that may prompt premature births, birth absconds, and hereditary harms in babies. If your work expects you to manage such

hardware, you may utilize gadgets that help decrease radiation or look for an adjustment in the idea of work.

17. Exposure to X-beams, particularly stomach X-beams, expands the danger of birth deformities and diseases, for example, leukemia in babies further down the road.

18. Do not remain close to microwaves, they transmit non-ionizing radiation, and introduction to more elevated levels of these radiations may cause inward body warming. This could influence the creating embryo. A harmed microwave may likewise build the danger of higher vitality releases that could be risky.

19. Do not utilize an electric cover. They emanate low-level electromagnetic fields, which can be risky for the developing baby. Additionally, abstain from overheating as this may bring about expanded centre temperature.

20. Do not utilize a waterbed as the radiators used in them emanate indistinguishable electric fields from electric covers.

21. Do not drink faucet water in early pregnancy stages if the water in your area is inclined to contaminants. Drink treated water.

22. Avoid pressure, particularly at work. It can influence your safe framework and increment the possibility of diseases prompting preterm labour.

23. Do not open yourself to pesticides, including herbicides, bug sprays, and fungicides. They can have an assortment of impacts on your hatchling, including unnatural birth cycle and preterm birth. If you can't stay away from introduction, wear a face cover.

24. Avoid exhaust from family cleaning items, paints, thinners, and so on. They contain solvents, which on inward breath increment the danger of unnatural birth cycle and birth surrenders. On the off chance that you can't stay away from introduction, wear a face cover.

25. Ensure that your body temperature isn't above 101°F as it tends to be conceivably risky for your creating baby. The body temperature ascends during influenza, strenuous exercises, and fever.

26. Ensure great individual cleanliness to avoid contracting illnesses, for example, herpes as it could prompt serious wellbeing intricacies in babies during delivery. In uncommon cases, it can likewise cause an unnatural birth cycle during the first trimester.

With such vast numbers of 'don'ts,' you may be thinking if there is whatever you can do during pregnancy. The appropriate response is yes.

Activities When Pregnant

Other than eating healthy, there is a lot of activities while pregnant. Check our trimester-wise plan for the day.

BELLY PHOTO HERE : 1-3 months

First trimester: Your primary daily agenda

This rundown encourages you to monitor activities in the first trimester – from pregnancy affirmation to remaining solid and picking a child name.

1. Test And Confirm Pregnancy

Utilizing home pregnancy tests, you can test your pregnancy precisely in seven days after you miss your period. This is two weeks post ovulation. If the test outcome is equivocal, sit tight for one more week and retake the test.

2. Find out About Health Insurance

Get some answers concerning medical coverage plans for pre-birth care and delivery costs. Numerous online destinations can assist you with this. If you are a working proficient, you could check with your organization's advantages division or the medical coverage organization.

3. Pick A Healthcare Provider

On the off chance that you have just picked your primary care physician or a birthing assistant, you are good to go. If not, you should search for one. Your loved ones can assist you with finding a medicinal services expert. Check how close or far they are, and whether they are under your medical coverage plan. If conceivable, meet a couple of them to check whether they are a solid match.

4. Get The Prenatal Appointment

Before seeing medicinal services professional, set yourself up by taking note of down the first day of your last period, and a rundown of inquiries to pose to your primary care physician. Get some answers concerning any illnesses or clutters in your and your significant other's families, and talk about them with your primary care physician.

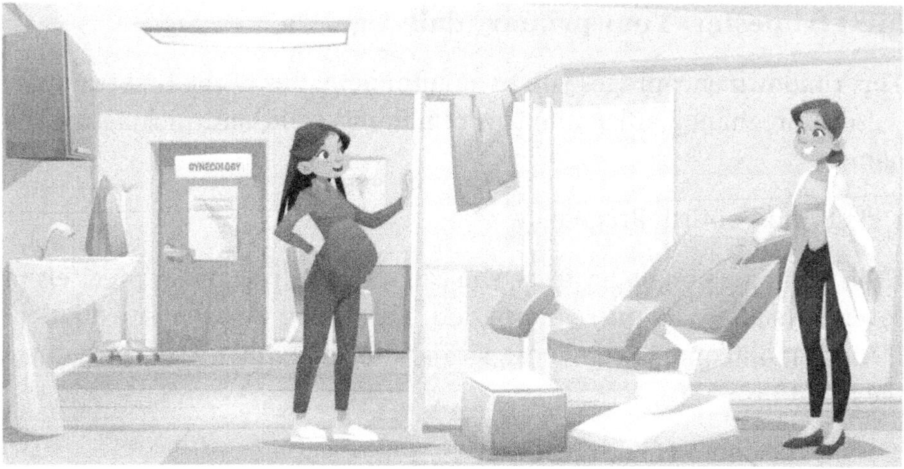

PRENATAL APPOINTMENTS

DATE	WK	WT	QUESTIONS FOR DOCTOR	NOTES

5. Educate About Medications

Most medications, including over-the-counter ones, are undependable during pregnancy. If you are on any meds, check with the specialist on the off chance that you can keep taking them or not. Notice the nutrients, herbs, or different enhancements that you have been seeking.

6. Time To Shed Your Habits

Stop smoking, liquor, and cutoff caffeine admission. They could cause premature labour and numerous pregnancy-related issues.

7. Eat Healthily

Counting a solid and adjusted diet can give all the necessary supplements that you and you infant require. Get some answers concerning nourishments you ought to and ought not to eat.

8. Handle Morning Sickness

Morning affliction keeps going the whole first trimester. On the off chance that it is mellow, at that point you can pursue straightforward estimates, for example, eating little and incessant suppers and adhering to tasteless nourishments. On the off chance that your condition is extreme, at that point you should converse with your expert right away.

9. Better Sleeping Habits

You might be increasingly drained or depleted during your first trimester as your body is changing following hormonal variances. Hit the sack early and rest more than you generally do. Unwind however much as could be expected by tuning in to relieving music or perusing a book.

10. Get ready To Announce Your Pregnancy

A few moms may declare pregnancy promptly, while some hold up until the subsequent trimester to preclude unnatural birth cycle. Additionally, you might need to postpone the declaration if there are pregnancy complexities or your activity is strenuous.

11. Pursue The Baby's Development

Buy into pregnancy pamphlets, so you will realize what's going on in your body and how your child is creating.

12. Start Taking Belly Pictures

Snap your photo consistently utilizing your appearance in a mirror or have somebody take it for you. You can see the improvement, and you will value these recollections sometime down the road. To have awesome pictures, wear a similar outfit, remain similarly situated, and have the same posture.

13. Grow Good Dressing Habits

Pick maternity bras as they offer great help. Additionally, like to purchase maternity briefs and swimsuits for additional solace.

14. Have Safe Sex

You might be excessively worn out, queasy, and moody. In any case, if you feel sensual, you can include in intercourse, as it won't hurt your child. The amniotic sac, solid uterine muscles, and thickened bodily fluid attachment will monitor the infant. Your primary care physician may request that you avoid sex in the first trimester.

15. Converse with Your Partner About Parenting

You can attempt one exploratory writing exercise here. Every one of you makes a rundown of how your mom and father parented you when you were a youngster. When you are done, choose which practices would increase the value of the infant's life and help you in bringing up your youngster decidedly.

16. Spending limit For The Baby

Consider how you can deal with the infant's costs – garments, nourishment, toys, diapers, and more child stuff. Check where you can trim your financial limit and think about profiting for utilizing it for your child.

17. Search For Baby Name Options

You may as of now have a couple of names at the top of the priority list, yet you would be astonished by the number of kinds there are to pick child names from.

18. Get Vaccinated Against Rubella (German measles)

Rubella can prompt premature deliveries and fetal variations from the norm during pregnancy. Get immunized before origination to evade the hazard.

MY FEELINGS AND THOUGHTS – 1° TRIMESTER

What went wrong? ______________________________

____

____

____

What was the positive side? ______________________________

____

____

____

____

List the beautiful and ugly emotions you experienced: _____

_____

Vote for myself: _____ Vote for my boyfriend: _____

5 weeks BABY IS THE SIZE OF A apple seed	6 weeks BABY IS THE SIZE OF A sweet pea	7 weeks BABY IS THE SIZE OF A blueberry	8 weeks BABY IS THE SIZE OF A raspberry
9 weeks BABY IS THE SIZE OF A strawberry	10 weeks BABY IS THE SIZE OF A prune	11 weeks BABY IS THE SIZE OF A lime	12 weeks BABY IS THE SIZE OF A plum
13 weeks BABY IS THE SIZE OF A peach	14 weeks BABY IS THE SIZE OF A lemon	15 weeks BABY IS THE SIZE OF A orange	16 weeks BABY IS THE SIZE OF A avocado

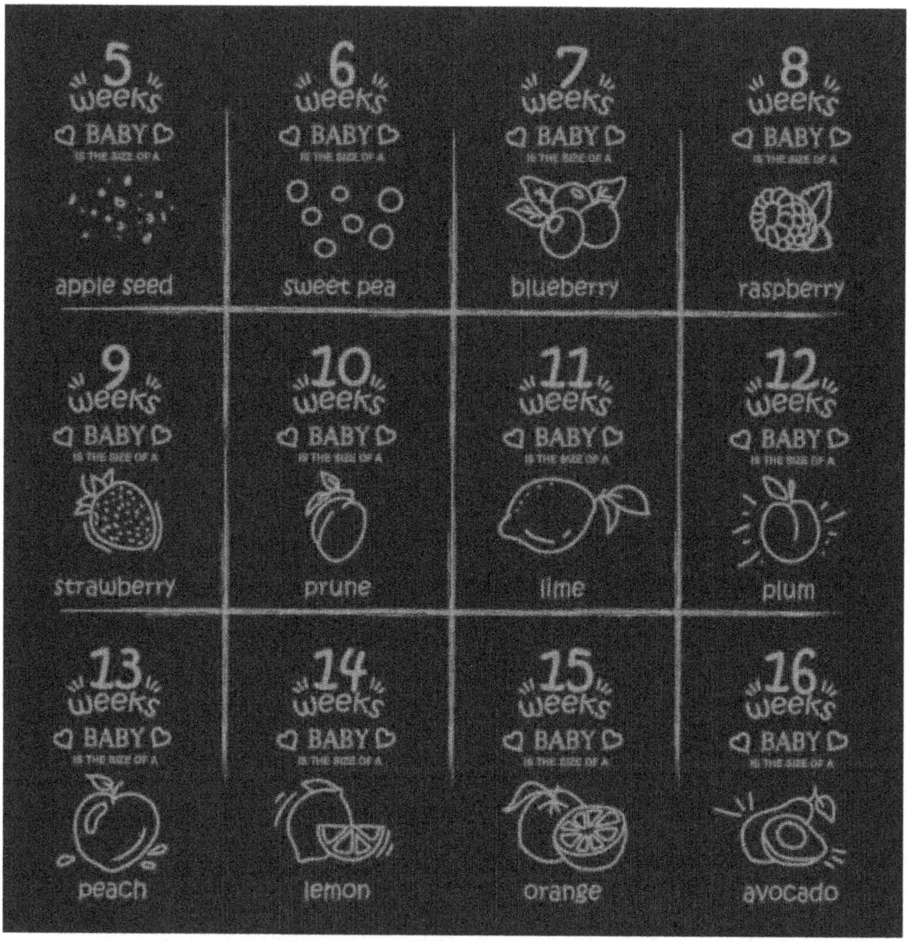

Second trimester: Your fundamental plan for the day

The second-trimester list encourages you to monitor everything from pre-birth tests to maternity leave and arranging a babymoon.

1. Pre-birth Visits And Tests

You should visit your professional once, like clockwork, except if there is any difficulty that calls for more tests than expected. You will have blood tests, screening tests, belly size estimations, and you can likewise observe the baby in the ultrasound checks.

2. Track Baby Development

Buy into pamphlets to see how your infant is creating. You can likewise download applications that assist you with knowing step by step or week-by-week child advancement and offer you essential guidance. Be that as it may, if all else fails, contact a medicinal service proficient.

3. Shop For Maternity Clothes

Maternity garments give you solace and let your body inhale forcefully. As your knock begins to appear (from 12 to 18 weeks), you will require several clothes that keep you calm. Along these lines, it bodes well to purchase the same number of as you need.

4. Choose A Professional Doula (Labor Coach)

Enlisting a prepared labour mentor or doula, who can help you during labour. She can offer you enthusiastic help and deal with your non-medicinal perspectives. The subsequent trimester is the best time to begin the hunt.

5. Saturate Your Belly

Applying a mellow moisturizer on your belly won't just diminish the stretch imprints, however, will likewise cut down the irritation. In any case, check with your primary care physician before utilizing a salve to guarantee that it is sans compound and doesn't hurt you or your infant.

6. Infant's Sex

Kid or young lady? An ultrasound can distinguish your child's sex. In any case, check if your nation enables you to take sexual orientation assurance tests. Likewise, ensure that you need to know the child's sexual orientation. You could generally pause and appreciate the amazement.

7. Record Your Pregnancy Dreams

You will recall a large portion you had always wanted because of the unpredictable rest cycle. Visit awakening to pee, leg cramps, spinal pain, acid reflux, and fretful leg disorder can upset your rest cycle in this trimester. Scribble down your fantasies and offer them with your accomplice. They can gain experiences and can be enjoyable.

BELLY PHOTO HERE : 3-6 months

8. Look-Into Childbirth Classes

Start your hunt immediately. Your emergency clinic gives you the classes, or you may select for a particular type someplace. For an in-person labour class, you can check with your emergency clinic or visit the International Childbirth Education Association part registry. On the off chance that conceivable, go to a level to get first-hand understanding.

9. Plan Your Finances

Put resources into protections. There will be new monetary duties be it the child's equations, diapers or sending them to class sometime down the road. You could visit gatherings, converse with loved ones, and get data on the sort of commercial ventures you should make.

8. Look-Into Childbirth Classes

Start your hunt immediately. Your emergency clinic gives you the classes, or you may select for a particular type someplace. For an in-person labour class, you can check with your emergency clinic or visit the International Childbirth Education Association part registry. On the off chance that conceivable, go to a level to get first-hand understanding.

9. Plan Your Finances

Put resources into protections. There will be new monetary duties be it the child's equations, diapers or sending them to class sometime down the road. You could visit gatherings, converse with loved ones, and get data on the sort of commercial ventures you should make.

10. Set up Your Older Child

On the off chance that you have more established youngsters, set them up for the new infant. Inform them concerning their diaper days, take them to pre-birth visits, make the new infant's room ahead of time so your kid becomes accustomed to the thought and continue conversing with them about the new kin.

11. Set up Your Pets

Pets likewise require particular pre-infant readiness. You can get nearby mentors for your pets, or allude to books, online recordings, or articles to see how to prepare your pet(s). Likewise, consider enlisting a pooch walker or pet sitter to make your lower your weight.

12. Get some answers concerning Childcare Centers

On the off chance that you intend to keep your infant in a childcare focus, start looking into different childcare focuses in your general vicinity. This should begin from the get-go to guarantee you settle on an educated choice.

13. Keep up Oral Hygiene

Clean teeth are an unquestionable requirement during pregnancy. If you have astounding oral wellbeing, you are less inclined to contract oral diseases and cavities during and after pregnancy.

14. Observe Mid-Pregnancy

At 20 weeks of pregnancy, you are part of the way through. Make it an occasion by going for a pedicure, pre-birth back rub, or wearing another outfit that pops your infant knock. Spend time with your accomplice, family, and companions and appreciate the stage.

15. Rest On Your Side

Rest on your side and not on the back. Rest to your left hand as it improves blood course along with the placenta and diminishes expanding. You can utilize a cushion under your hips, beneath your back, or potentially between your legs for an agreeable position.

16. Plan Your Maternity Leave

This is the point at which you should choose when to take your maternity leave. Check with your organization's human asset office. Ensure you comprehend the leave plan and perceive how well you can design your assignments and undertakings.

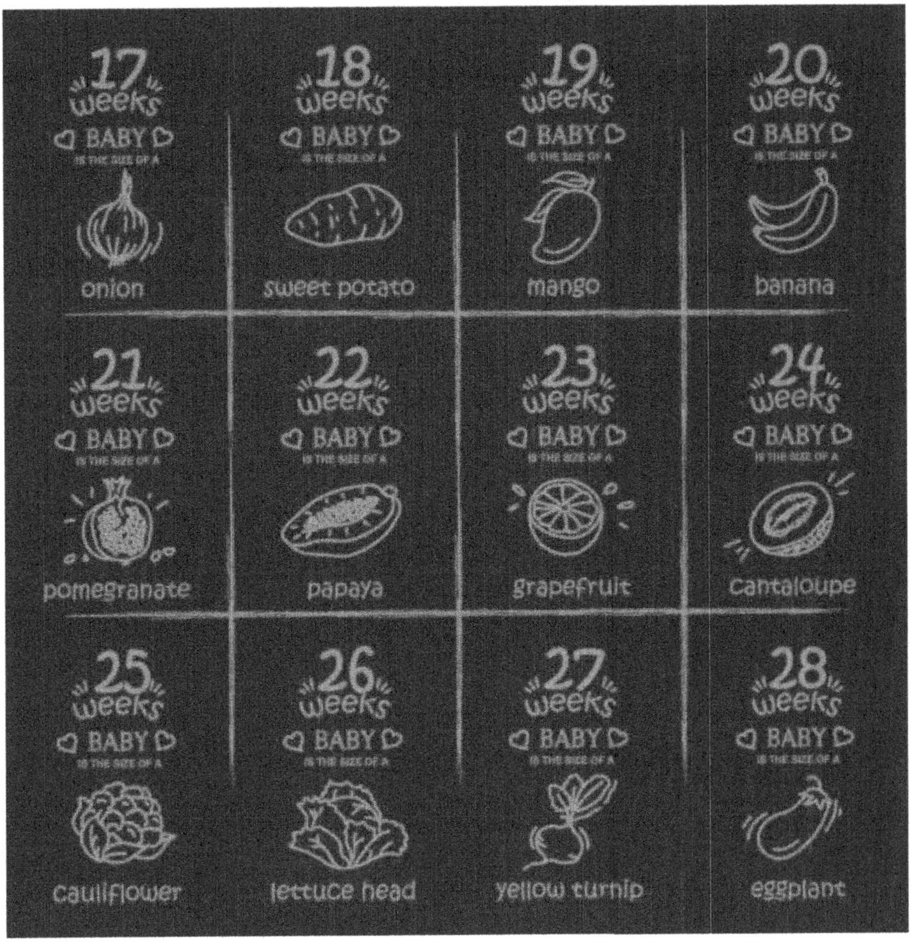
17 weeks
BABY
onion
18 weeks
BABY
sweet potato
19 weeks
BABY
mango
20 weeks
BABY
banana
21 weeks
BABY
pomegranate
22 weeks
BABY
papaya
23 weeks
BABY
grapefruit
24 weeks
BABY
cantaloupe
25 weeks
BABY
cauliflower
26 weeks
BABY
lettuce head
27 weeks
BABY
yellow turnip
28 weeks
BABY
eggplant

17. Check Your Fingerings

As your pregnancy advances, you can see your fingers growing. If you feel the rings are snug, take them off at an early stage before they stall out. On the off chance that you would prefer not to leave behind it, take it off and put it to your chain, so it stays near your heart.

18. Plan A Babymoon

In your subsequent trimester, you will be free from morning affliction, and feel like yourself once more. Since the up and coming third trimester expedites weariness once more, presently is the ideal time for you to design an outing.

19. Incline toward A Baby Shower

Even though moms-to-be don't usually have a child shower, you can have your family member, accomplice, or a companion have it for you. You can likewise share your inclinations on the list of people to attend, topics, and games.

20. Home Improvement Projects

You should begin setting up your new child's space, sort out storerooms, assess things, and fix the house to make it infant safe before the infant shows up. Look for your accomplice's assistance in the undertaking.

21. Allot Some Partner-Time

Alongside the child arrangements, invest significant energy for your accomplice and praise the event. Probably the ideal ways are to observe things you love about one another, take sentimental walks, or tell your accomplice how he can turn into an incredible parent.

22. Well-Balanced Diet

You require around 340 extra calories for each day in your subsequent trimester. Make a diagram of essential nourishments you can take and glue it in your storeroom or on the fridge. Note what you have included for that day, and add any extra nourishments to the night menu. In any case, keep it light and sound.

MY FEELINGS AND THOUGHTS – 2° TRIMESTER

What went wrong? ____

____

____

What was the positive side? ____

____

____

Do you have anything learned from mistakes? ____________________

____

List the beautiful and ugly emotions you experienced: ____________

____

Vote for myself: ____________ Vote for my boyfriend: ____________

Third trimester: Your fundamental plan for the day

This rundown can assist you with monitoring all your third-trimester exercises and undertakings – from following child's developments to stocking up infant's garments and adapting up too late pregnancy butterflies.

1. Know about Baby's Movements

Your specialist can show you how the child's kicks. Perceive your child's boots, rolls, and jerks, and illuminate the specialist if you notice any lessening in developments. Fewer developments can be because of any hidden condition that your specialist may make sense of.

2. Pre-birth Visits And Tests

You will have a pre-birth test two times per week from week 28 to week 36, and afterwards once per week until labour. You will have distinctive physical tests, pregnancy tests, and exchanges with your specialist about approaching birth.

3. More On Baby Care Classes

Aside from labour class, you ought to likewise consider taking up lessons on infant care, nursing, and newborn child cardiopulmonary revival (CPR). A few emergency clinics offer them, or you can approach your expert for a proposal.

4. Get ready For Nursing

You ought to learn as much as you can about breastfeeding your infant. Converse with nursing moms and specialists, read articles and books to find out additional or take a breastfeeding class.

5. Pick A Pediatrician

Your infant will have their first specialist's visit soon after delivery. Make a rundown of the considerable number of pediatricians and family specialists from your companions, family, neighbours, and associates. At that point, make sense of the facility or zone that is advantageous for you, and mind how great the specialist is.

6. Plan for an impressive future

Would you like to remain with your child regularly or low maintenance? Will you have any strict function after labour? Do you need to bank your infant's rope blood? These might be some significant choices to consider this time.

7. Set up A Baby Gear

You may take your accomplice's or companion's assistance. Start purchasing beds, surreys, lodgings, buggies, and then some. Organizing these now can make your life simpler after labour.

8. Set up The Baby's Bed

Den or bassinet, whatever you decide for your infant, it is essential to pursue the set rules to bring down the odds of unexpected baby passing disorder (SIDS).

9. Converse with Your Baby

From the third trimester, your child can hear your voice, so conversing with them can help in holding better. You can peruse a book, paper, or offer your desires with your kid. This additionally enables your infant to create language abilities.

10. Adapting To Labor Pain

Each labour is unique, and each lady's involvement in the pain is extraordinary. It is a great idea to find out about delivery choices, regardless of whether to have prompted labour or special delivery and knowing their advantages and disadvantages to pick better.

11. Become familiar with The Stages Of Labor

Labour is isolated into three significant stages, and together it goes on for quite a long time along. Also, if it is your first pregnancy, it takes additional time. Finding out pretty much this would set you up for labour.

12. Make A Birth Plan

This is a route for you to impart yours wants to your primary care physicians or maternity specialists who deal with you during labour. It causes them to comprehend what sort of job you would need to have.

Things may not go as you wish, however making an arrangement can assist you with settling on better choices in regards to labour.

13. Make sense of Helpers

You might be needing a family help after your infant is conceived. Cause a rundown of individuals who to can assist you with the trip and set assignments. Assignments could be bringing you dinners, getting arrangements, dealing with more established youngsters, tidying up, and different errands.

BELLY PHOTO HERE : 6-7 months

14. Observe Your Belly

Remember your developing knock by gracing it with pretty plans, (for example, face paints), getting henna, or making a belly cast. You may likewise get proficient pictures painted on your belly. Be that as it may, recall, whatever you do, keep away from manufactured hues as they could be dangerous. Utilize just natural shades and check for allergens.

15. Gather Your Hospital Bag

You may start giving birth and scramble for delivery whenever. Consequently, it is always a smart thought to gather your sack well ahead of time. Take your accomplice's assistance – protection cards, open to dressing, toiletries, outfits, portable charger, and that's only the tip of the iceberg.

16. Clean Your House

Take the assistance of any relative or a companion to have your home cleaned before the child's introduction to the world. This would guarantee a protected and clean condition for your child when you return home from the medical clinic with your infant.

17. Load Up On Household Supplies

Stock up the washroom, fridge, prescription, toiletries with enough supplies. Get clean cushions, shampoos, and additional sets of innerwear. Additionally, make a point to have enough infant supplies.

18. Introduce Car Seat For The Baby

Get ready to have a child vehicle seat with the goal that it gets simpler to drive your infant around. You may locate the best items via looking through on the web or conversing with your primary care physician and companions.

19. Approaches To Announce Baby's Arrival

Make a rundown of approaches to tell individuals after the infant's delivery. Some like to post reports via web-based networking media while others incline toward calling, messaging, or messaging. Set up a rundown of telephone numbers and email delivers to whom you need to pass the uplifting news.

20. Know about Late-Pregnancy Issues

There could be explicit pregnancy difficulties that may spring up in your third trimester, for example, preeclampsia and unexpected labour. Keep a watch of the side effects to call your PCP right away.

21. Adapt To Late-Pregnancy Fears

There might be numerous things that can make you anxious as your due date approaches. Fears of labour pain, the wellbeing of your new child, and the idea of how well you would alter as another mother are healthy. You should attempt to conquer them by following unwinding procedures, checking with different moms, and conversing with your social insurance supplier.

22. Expertise Your Body Changes Post-Delivery

Some first-time moms alarm in the wake of seeing their baby blues body. Even though it might be challenging to acknowledge changes, attempt to comprehend that it took you nine months to get you there, the body would bob back with time.

23. Try not to Worry If You Are Overdue

You might be concerned if you don't convey near your due date. This is very normal, and your human services professionals will assist you with drugs and methods to start labour.

These trimester-wise dos will make your pregnancy simple, and post-pregnancy lose as you have just arranged your strategy.

MY FEELINGS AND THOUGHTS – 3° TRIMESTER

What went wrong? ____

____

What was the positive side? ____

____

____

List the beautiful and ugly emotions you experienced: __________

____

Hyphotetical names for the baby – I would like to call him: ______

____

My boyfriend instead: __________________ Common: ________

Vote for myself: __________ Vote for my boyfriend: ___________

What To Do In All Trimesters

Here is an extreme show you ought to pursue all through the pregnancy independent of the trimester.

1. Drink more water

You should drink around eight to ten glasses of liquids consistently. Convey a water bottle with you generally and taste in always. It maintains a strategic distance from drying out and forestalls urinary tract diseases. Additionally, check the shade of your pee. If it is dim yellow, you ought to drink more water. Clear pee shows you are very much hydrated.

2. Get customary therapeutic tests

Common medicinal assessments guarantee that you don't have any entanglements and issues during pregnancy.

3. Devour enough folic corrosive

By getting the RDA (suggested day by day stipend) of 0.4mg folic corrosive, you will bring down your infant's danger of neural cylinder abandons.

5. Incorporate pre-birth nutrients

Taking pre-birth nutrients will give the essential nutrition to both you and your infant. They likewise keep pregnancy difficulties under control.

6. Take a lot of protein

Satisfactory protein is essential for infant advancement and counteracts preeclampsia during pregnancy. The RDA of protein is 75 grams.

7. Eat and exercise

Your ordinary diet requires a lot of nutrients, minerals, proteins, fibre, and the sky is the limit from there. You ought to likewise exercise to keep up a perfect weight.

8. Get the necessary fat from the diet

Fat and cholesterol are fundamental for engrossing fat-dissolvable nutrients A, D, E, and K. They are imperative for stretchable skin and infant mental health. You may need to check with your professional about what fat nourishments to remember for your diet.

9. Perform kegel exercises

Frail kegel muscles add to pain during labour, delayed second stage, and untimely flexion of the child's head. Labour likewise debilitates the muscles and causes numerous distresses. You should, hence, do kegel exercises to evade every one of these issues.

10. Use houseplants

Attempt to have houseplants that are great at disposing of concealed synthetic substances at home. For example, arachnid plants are great at retaining formaldehyde.

11. Be cautious while voyaging

Find out about security works on during voyaging. You should be extra cautious, particularly when you are heading out to outside nations or are on long voyages.

12. Get data on conditions and therapeutic chronicles

On the off chance that you are now experiencing any condition or having a family ancestry of regenerative issues, carry them to your primary care physician's notification.

13. Include in some extending

Do extend exercises as it keeps your muscles from fixing, upgrades adaptability, and makes you feel loose and adaptable. 12. Get data on conditions and therapeutic chronicles

BELLY PHOTO HERE : 8-9 months

14. Take a power rest

You will get exhausted and may require 15 minutes rest to resuscitate yourself. Enjoy a reprieve, whether at work or at home. You could set short alerts on your telephone and sneak in a power rest.

15. Pack nutritional bites

Have some solid bites prepared at your home, handbag, vehicle, or work area, so it is anything but difficult to swallow them when you are ravenous. On the off chance that you feel disgusted, chomp on essential tidbits, (for example, wafers) to facilitate the inclination.

16. Unwinding method

Guided symbolism, profound breathing exercises, dynamic muscle unwinding, and pre-birth yoga help you to stay calm and advance great rest.

17. Go for a stroll

Taking a 15 to 20-minute walk each day can keep your vitality step up.

18. Incorporate pregnancy superfoods

Give your pregnancy a lift by devouring bright vegetables and natural products, salmon, yogurt, pecans, sweet potatoes, beans, and that's only the tip of the iceberg.

19. Note down pregnancy recollections

Keep up a proper diary or note down certain things about your pregnancy that kept your spirits high. You will cherish imparting them to your youngster sometime down the road.

20. Control your weight

Your expert will screen your weight at each pre-birth exam to guarantee that you are in a perfect weight territory.

21. Offer with your companion

If you have any feelings of dread, wants, and wishes, share them with your accomplice or companions.

22. Accomplish something bravo

Attempt to improve the adventure by going out to see a film, arranging a supper, getting a spa treatment, or whatever else you appreciate. In sort, spoil yourself.

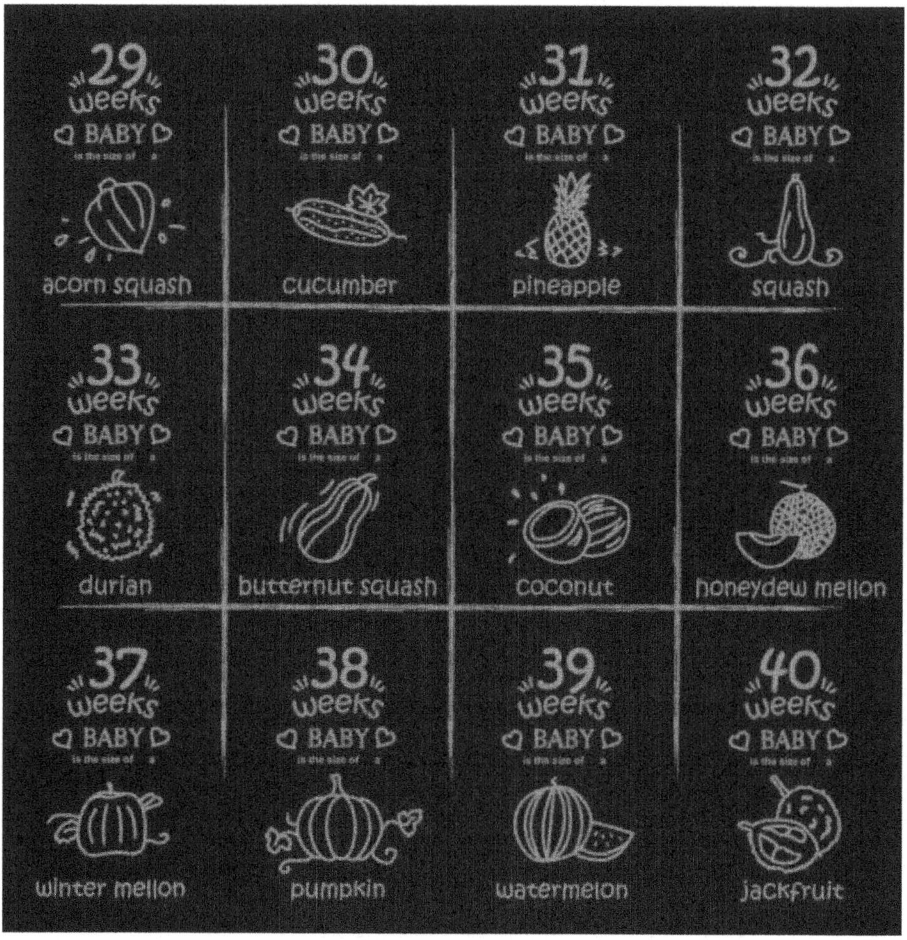

HISTORY OF THE CHILD - ECHOGRAPHS

Paste the photos

10th week

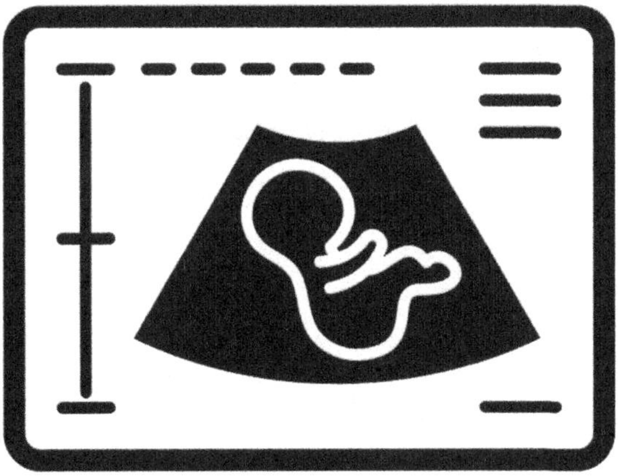

20th – 22th week

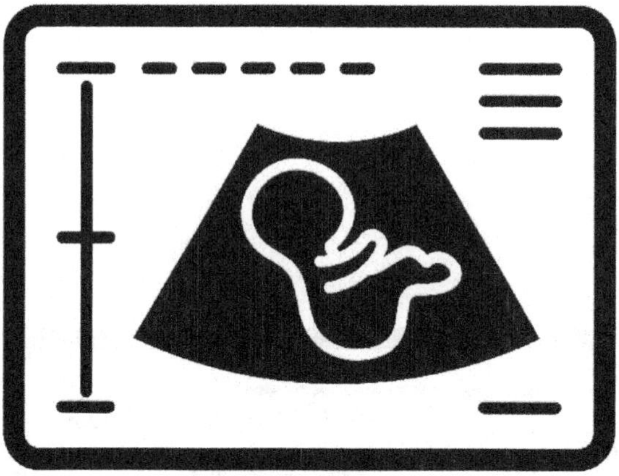

32th – 34th week

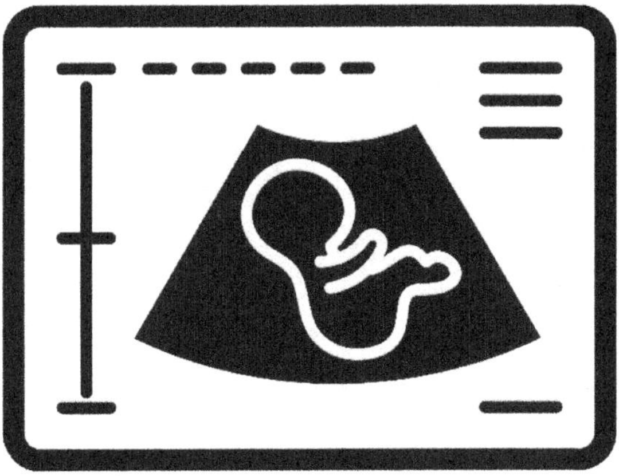

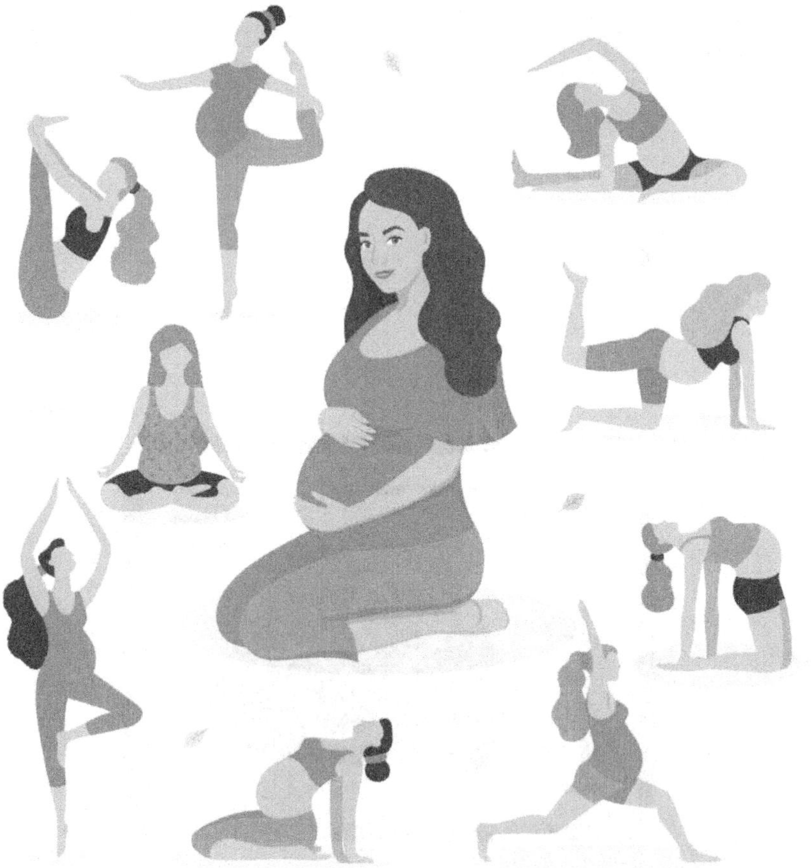

"Motherhood is the biggest gamble in the world. It is the glorious life force. It's huge and scary—it's an act of infinite optimism."

- *Gilda Radner*

CHAPTER THREE

WARNING SYMPTOMS THAT A PREGNANT WOMAN SHOULD NEVER IGNORE

Safe Sleeping Positions During First Trimester Of Pregnancy

Ladies feel tired during pregnancy, particularly during their first trimester, and require more rest than previously. The early pregnancy side effects like laziness, nervousness, queasiness, acid reflux, and noon can include outings, heartburn, and even eager leg disorder (RLS) may influence the rest designs. Be that as it may, a couple of way of life changes can improve your first-trimester rest to make you rest soundly.

Explanations for Lack Of Sleep During First Trimester

Your body experiences a lot of changes, which disturb your sound rest. As per the National Sleep Foundation (1998) Poll on Women and Sleep, 78% of ladies are accounted for to encounter rest aggravations during pregnancy than different times. Recorded beneath are the signs that hamper your rest in the early pregnancy organize.

1. Tired constantly:

You will feel exceptionally sluggish from the get-go in your pregnancy, particularly during the day. The ascent of progesterone hormone achieves this abrupt change in rest designs. This hormone controls the lady's regenerative cycle making you weary. The thermogenic (heat delivering) and balmy (rest prompting) impacts of progesterone lead to weariness and early rest beginning and cause you depleted, giving the bogus thought of influenza.

An exploration study found that in the first trimester, the absolute rest time increments is of low quality because of awakening always. There is additionally a decrease in profound rest when contrasted with pre-

pregnancy. Most ladies griped of laziness, weakness, and discouragement.

2. Distress with body changes:

Your delicate and sore breasts make it hard for you to rest comfortably. If you want to lie on your stomach, it will be less agreeable as your knock fires appearing.

Arrangement: Try sleeping on your side, which is a perfect situation for your infant's sustenance. Likewise, ensure you wear an appropriate bra to suit your developing breasts. You can wear an agreeable games bra or maternity rest bra while sleeping and utilize a body pad to help your irritated nipples. On the off chance that breast irritation is upsetting your rest, your primary care physician may recommend acetaminophen, FDA Pregnancy Category C medicate.

3. Urge to always pee:

Progesterone hormone is likewise mostly liable for the endless inclination to pee. The inhibitory impacts of the hormones on smooth muscles invigorate the desire. With the advancing pregnancy, the developing knock will likewise put weight on the bladder and subsequently increment the pee recurrence. You will be awakening as often as possible to diminish your bladder, and it will, consequently, upset your sleep at evenings.

Arrangement: If you are burnt out on the restroom visits, do whatever it takes not to remove the liquid admission. Instead, drink more during the daytime and less before bedtime. Additionally, cut off caffeine drinks like tea, espresso, and cola.

4. Sickness:

Morning affliction is very reasonable in the underlying 12 weeks of pregnancy, and most ladies create queasiness whenever of the day. It can likewise wake you up in the night, in this manner upsetting your rest. Queasiness is, for the most part, exacerbated by low glucose levels in pregnancy.

Arrangement: You can beat queasiness by attempting some homegrown cures or enhancements in the wake of counselling your PCP. Ginger is one excellent solution for beat this. Pressure point massage helps as well.

5. Indigestion:

Progesterone hormone shows loosening up consequences for everything in your body. It likewise loosens up the smooth muscles that are opening into your stomach from the throat. It is along these lines, permits stomach substance and acids stream once more into your throat, causing heartburn after your supper, disturbing your rest post supper.

Arrangement: You should give legitimate time for the nourishment to process before you rest. Eat gradually and monitor nourishments which can cause issues.

6. Stress and tension:

The first-trimester pregnancy is a blend of astonishments and enthusiasm, particularly for first-time moms. While acclimating to the physical and mental changes, a couple of ladies may feel extraordinary, and others dreadful. An investigation on first-time moms versus experienced moms demonstrated that the accomplished ladies had an extra 45 minutes to one hour of rest each night.

Arrangement: If you are excessively focused on, note down your sentiments in a book and take a stab at discovering methods. For instance, on the off chance that you are anxious about the delivery, you can pursue a labour class which helps facilitate your brain. You should settle down before bedtime with mitigating exercises like having some warm milk, a warm shower, tuning in to loud music, or enjoying unwinding practices.

Best Sleeping Positions During First Trimester

How might you get that valuable rest while encountering all the above issues that disturb your rest?

1. Sleeping On Side (SOS):

Lying as an afterthought is far superior to sleeping on your front or back. Yet, the best sleeping position is on the left side. Resting on the privilege can create pressure on the liver and your PCP will request that you evade that. Left would be the best position as it keeps the developing uterus from applying pressure on the liver, enabling the embryo to get enough oxygen and supplements through the placenta. It additionally improves blood dissemination and decreases the vitality spent in drawing the ideal bloodstream for both mother and child.

You can interchange your situation to one side on the off chance that you dislike sleeping on the left for quite a while. You should don't hesitate to substitute starting with one hand then onto the next, however, ensure you don't rest on the appropriate for quite a while. Sleeping on one side with your knees, bowed is the most agreeable position.

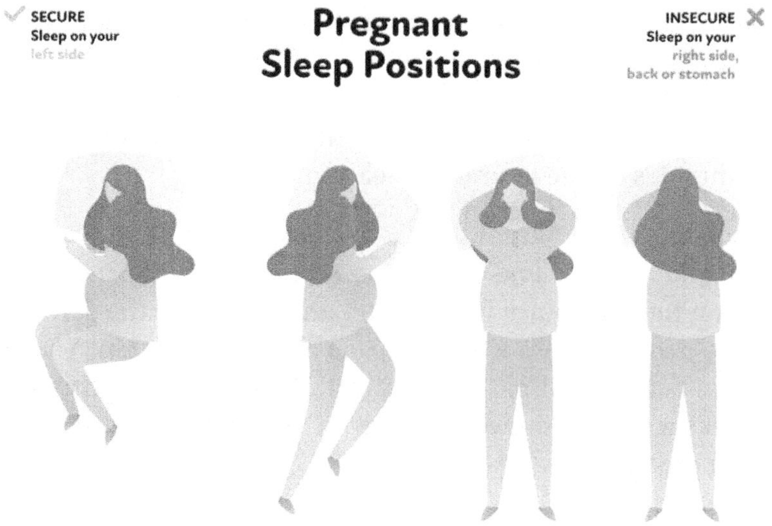
SECURE
Sleep on your
left side
Pregnant
Sleep Positions
INSECURE
Sleep on your
right side,
back or stomach

2. Sleeping On Back:

In the underlying phases of pregnancy, you can decide to rest on the back if you are utilized to that position. Nonetheless, as the pregnancy progresses, you ought to abstain from a lying level on your back. It is because the developing uterus applies pressure on your back muscles, spine, significant veins, which in this manner change the bloodstream in your body and child.

Sleeping on the back will likewise give you muscle pains, growing, and hemorrhoids. The position can cause a drop in the circulatory strain levels, which may prompt dazedness. For certain ladies, it can cause a rise in the circulatory strain and may prompt snoring and inevitably rest apnea (shallows breaths while sleeping). Sleeping on your back, in a half-sitting situation by taking the help of a couple of cushions is okay and help those experiencing acid reflux. The first trimester is simply the correct time to get changed by sleeping on your left side, which is the perfect position.

Does Lack Sleep Harm Your Baby?

It won't hurt your child as rest issues are typical during pregnancy. However, you ought to tune in to your body when it requests that you rest or back off. Less stay in bed early pregnancy can expand the danger of pre-eclampsia and hypertension in moms.

Sleeping Aids During Pregnancy

Tranquillizers help in offering you agreeable and sound rest, particularly during your first and third trimesters which are great times of pregnancy.

1. Cushions:

Cushions can assist you with maintaining a strategic distance from restless evenings. For back and belly support – Tuck one cushion between your bowed knees to help your lower back. It will likewise make your side sleeping position agreeable. You can utilize a full-body cushion for your return or front. It gives you the correct help while lying on your side. You can attempt different pillows, either usually utilized ones or those accessible explicitly for pregnancy use. You may utilize body-length, U or C-molded pillows, or wedge-formed pads to help your belly or chest.

On the off chance that you are experiencing acid reflux: You can keep one additional pad underneath your head to lift it while you are sleeping. It helps in keeping the stomach acids set up because of gravity as opposed to letting those head out back to the throat.

If you have hip pain: If you experience body pains or hip pain while lying as an afterthought, a solid sleeping cushion will help. An egg-box froth sleeping pad can be put on your regular bedding. It will bolster your middle and appendages, and give you agreeable rest without hurting hips.

2. Nourishment and drink:

What you eat and drink, and when you take them, will likewise influence your rest quality. Maintain a strategic distance from caffeine and sugar, which are the regular rest snatchers. A glass of warm milk before bedtime is a deeply rooted solution for proper rest.

For low glucose: If cerebral pains, awful dreams, or extraordinary perspiring upset your rest, you might be experiencing low glucose levels. You can take protein pressed snacks, for example, nutty spread, egg, or turkey, before bedtime to keep glucose levels high during rest.

For sickness: Nausea can create due to a vacant stomach. In this manner, you ought to have a light tidbit containing sugars and proteins before bedtime. Great choices incorporate – a half sandwich with milk, high-protein oat with milk, or a high protein smoothie. You can eat some tasteless, dry tidbits like pretzels, rice cakes, and saltines if you happen to wake up feeling sick.

For acid reflux and heartburn: Avoid taking huge suppers before bedtime or late in the day. Sleeping on a full stomach will decline the condition.

3. Booked rest:

Arranging your rest time is likewise crucial during pregnancy. You should have to take rests at whatever point conceivable. The best time is somewhere in the range of two and four p.m. You can break them into two 30-minutes snoozes instead of one long 2-hours rest. Try not to take excessive liquids after six p.m. as they lessen nighttime washroom visits.

Unwinding Techniques For Better Pregnancy Sleep

You can likewise attempt the accompanying necessary and time-tried procedures to loosen up your muscles, quiet your brain, and rest adequately.

1. Yoga and extending:

They help you unwind, conditioned your body and make it adaptable all through the pregnancy. There are numerous fitness centres and recreation centres that teach yoga and extending preparing to pregnant ladies. You can likewise build up your system that includes basic moves for neck and bears, back and midriff calves and hamstrings. Doing them during the day and before heading to sleep will assist you with nodding off rapidly. Remember that you have to carefully pursue the rules given by your coach or specialist while doing any exercise during the first trimester. If you are awkward doing a given posture, at that point, stay away from it.

2. Profound relaxing:

Profound and cadenced breathing will bring down pulse, ease muscle pressure, and advance great rest.

3. Back rub:

Back rub helps in loosening up the muscles that are inclined to pressure and consequently offering great rest. You can likewise get an expert back rub by talking about the alternative with your primary care physician before arranging it. Another incredible route is to get a hand, foot, or neck rub from your accomplice.

4. Dynamic muscle unwinding:

This is a necessary unwinding procedure that encourages you to rest sufficiently. The primary thought is to discharge the fixed muscles by straining and loosening up them. Lie on the bed or floor. Concentrate on one gathering of muscles, and have a go at switching back and forth among both way sides. Firstly, tense and discharge hand and lower arm muscles, trailed by an upper arm, face and jaw, shoulder, back, thighs until you go to your feet.

5. Guided symbolism:

It quiets your restless personality and advances a profound rest. Close your eyes and think about an excellent and loosening up place. Or then again consider skimming mists along the water edge. Have a go at envisioning each moment detail, for example, smell, surface, shading, sound, taste, and so forth. You need to envision yourself, so it connects with your brain in a virtual world, and it redirects your consideration from the idea of restlessness.

Additionally, don't decide to exercise inside four hours of rest time. It will fire up you and upset your rest cycle. Instead, you can burn some calories in the day and early at night.

Would you be able to rest on your stomach in the first trimester?

For whatever length of time that you are open to sleeping on your stomach, you are allowed to rest so. In any case, you will think that it's difficult to rest on the stomach with the developing belly. This position is additionally known to remove the blood supply to the embryo, and can prompt wooziness and queasiness and consequently, it is ideal for maintaining a strategic distance from it.

What amount would it be a good idea for you to rest in the first trimester?

Grown-ups, for the most part, require a normal of seven to nine hours of complete rest each night. In any case, with the requests of pregnancy on a lady's body, you may require more rest during the first trimester. The sleeping hours may change from one lady to the other. Be that as it may, you ought to tune in to your body and give it rest when expected to die down rest aggravations.

Progesterone During Pregnancy: Level High Or Too Low?

Mood swings, nourishment desires, tiredness, and morning ailment – these are the first pregnancy indications activated by the hormonal changes in the body. Progesterone is one of the essential pregnancy hormones that assume a first job in the lady's body. Through the nine months, the degrees of progesterone continue fluctuating, and that outcomes in a few physical changes. Excited about realizing what happens when the progesterone levels rise or fall?

What Is Progesterone?

Progesterone is a hormone that controls delicate cycle and richness. It is discharged by the corpus luteum or the transitory endocrine organ that is shaped in the ovary of the female body. The hormone is delivered after ovulation or after the release of eggs from the ovary. If you imagine, progesterone helps the coating of the uterus to plan for implantation and afterwards keeps up it all through the pregnancy. In the fact that you don't consider, the organ separates and decreases the progesterone levels, bringing about the monthly cycle.

How Does Progesterone Help Before And During Pregnancy?

Progesterone assumes a first job in getting ready and keeping up the endometrium (layer covering of the uterus), along these lines helping the hatchling's endurance.

• During the luteal stage (the stage after ovulation in a menstrual cycle), the hormone advances the development of veins and actuates the discharge of the endometrial organ. This thickens the covering of the uterus to acknowledge and support the treated egg.

• In the growth time frame, progesterone elevates unwinding of muscles to avert compressions. During pregnancy, the hormone makes an appropriate situation for the baby to develop.

• Even during lactation, progesterone invigorates milk-delivering cells.

Progesterone assumes an indispensable job in the working of the lady's conceptive cycle. Additionally, progesterone impacts endometrium secretory changes, looks after pregnancy, and decreases uterine contractility. Consequently, it is fundamental to have adjusted degrees of progesterone in the body: depending on your age, ask your doctor for an opinion on a possible supplement.

Estrogen and Progesterone

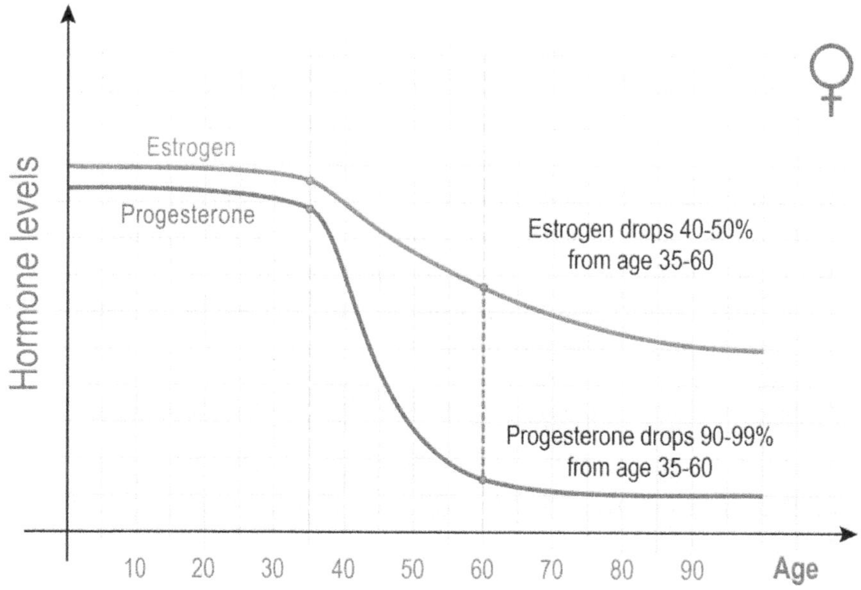

What Happens If Progesterone Levels Are High During Pregnancy?

Hormonal equalization is necessary for the body to work appropriately. At the point when progesterone levels ascend during pregnancy, you could encounter specific manifestations, for example, tiredness, swelling, uneasiness, and diminished sex drive. In uncommon cases, there could be unfavourable impacts on decidualization (changes to endometrial cells) and endometrial receptivity. The degrees of progesterone, in any case can be overseen and kept up ideally.

How To Keep Progesterone In Control?

A reliable way of life that incorporates regular exercise, a well-adjusted diet, less low-quality nourishment, no smoking or liquor, and legitimate rest could help in adjusting the progesterone levels in the body.

In some instances, progesterone levels could go low, and that isn't great.

What Happens If Progesterone Levels Are Too Low?

Low progesterone levels could be an issue on the off chance that you are attempting to get pregnant or when you are pregnant. Sporadic periods, cerebral pains, and mood swings are the manifestations you'll encounter when the progesterone is low in your body.

At the point when the body doesn't discharge enough progesterone, there could be estrogen (another pregnancy hormone) predominance that could bring about side effects, for example, misery, weight concerns, breast delicacy, and even gallbladder issues. While there are certain dangers of low progesterone levels, there are additionally approaches to bring the hormone levels up to commonality.

What Are The Different Forms Of Progesterone?

Given the progesterone levels in your body, the specialist will recommend the type of progesterone supplement you should take. Enlighten the specialist concerning any hypersensitivities or wellbeing conditions you have before making a progesterone supplement.

1. Vaginal gel: It is endorsed as a piece of richness treatment for ladies who are attempting to get pregnant. It is likewise recommended when ladies have sporadic or no periods because of low progesterone levels. The gel should be put away at room temperature. Ensure you counsel your primary care physician before utilizing any over-the-counter (OTC) progesterone vaginal gel.

2. Vaginal suppository: This medication is aggravated by the drug specialist and requirements exceptional consideration for utilizing. It is endorsed to counteract preterm delivery or premature labor in pregnant ladies, or for ladies with specific conditions, for example, corpus luteum deficiency, bringing about low progesterone levels. This ought to be put away in a fridge.

3. Vaginal addition: It is a tablet that contains a micronized manufactured type of progesterone hormone, which is made for the vaginal organization.

4. Progesterone infusion: It is endorsed to treat irregular uterine draining or menstrual periods because of unevenness in progesterone. The injection is just recommended and given by a specialist.

The utilization, dose, and the span of any of these types of progesterone are endorsed by the specialist and ought to be pursued precisely. Talk about with your primary care physician and pick an alternative that is protected and helpful for you.

When Should You Discontinue Taking Progesterone During Pregnancy?

The course of progesterone as infusions, supplements, suppositories, or different methods ought to be as endorsed by the specialist. As the explanation behind progesterone supplementation is diverse for each lady, the length of treatment would likewise be extraordinary. A few specialists propose ceasing the progesterone supplementation somewhere in the range of 9 and 12 weeks of pregnancy.

Are There Any Side Effects Of Synthesized Forms Of Progesterone?

Indeed, even though progesterone supplements are viewed as protected, there could be explicit reactions, for example,

• Change in pee and stool shading

• Nausea, mood swings, and misfortune or increment in craving

• Abnormal vaginal dying

• Stomach cramps, back pain, or chest pain

• Swelling or pain in the arms or legs

• Changes in visual perception

• Yellowing of skin or eyes

• Tiredness, perplexity, wooziness, and inconvenience talking or comprehension

• Allergic responses, for example, itching, rashes, and expanding of tongue, lips, or even face.

It is smarter to counsel your primary care physician, comprehend the symptoms, and afterward choose whether or not to take the progesterone supplements.

What Are The Safety And Precautionary Measures To Be Taken?

In a perfect world, the progesterone supplements are sheltered when taken according to the specialist's solution. In any case, if you have certain wellbeing conditions or sensitivities, you ought to maintain a strategic distance from them.

1. Let your primary care physician know whether the indications are extreme and disturbing you.

2. Don't utilize the enhancements for a drawn-out period as that may cause wellbeing inconveniences.

3. Let your primary care physician know whether you have any wellbeing condition, for example, coronary illness, liver ailment, vaginal dying, sorrow, or any hypersensitivities that progesterone may decline.

4. When progesterone is utilized to avert unexpected labor or as a piece of richness treatment, it is viewed as protected. Else, it ought not to be used during pregnancy or to diminish premenstrual disorder or disturbance or pain.

Continue perusing to realize the responses to some usually posed inquiries about progesterone levels during pregnancy.

Does progesterone consumption increment the possibility of premature labor?

No, progesterone is taken to help a healthy pregnancy. Notwithstanding, its utilization ought to be as indicated by the specialist's remedy. Never take any progesterone supplements without counseling the specialist first. The specialist can suggest the best variation and the measurements of progesterone that you should take contingent upon your condition.

Does taking progesterone cause birth surrenders?

No, proof doesn't recommend any connection among progesterone and birth abandons. A few examinations have indicated that taking progesterone causes no harmful impacts or innate incapacities in kids.

Could there be any pregnancy difficulties with progesterone use?

In a perfect world, there ought to be no intricacies with the utilization of progesterone supplements. Be that as it may, on account of hypersensitivities or certain wellbeing conditions, it is recommended that you keep away from its use.

Would I be able to take progesterone while breastfeeding?

Truly, progesterone may enter breast milk in little amounts. However, there is no damage to your child in any capacity. If you are still in question about progesterone and nursing, converse with your PCP. Progesterone assumes a significant job in supporting pregnancy. To keep up this present hormone's levels in the body, it is essential to be reliable and fit. Yet, if for reasons unknown, the hormone levels get tilted, counsel your primary care physician, and get treated in time.

Taking Folic Acid In Pregnancy

Folic corrosive or folate, which is alluded to as the 'pregnancy superhuman,' ought to be devoured by ladies when they get pregnant.

What Is Folic Acid?

Folic corrosive is a manufactured type of nutrient B9 found in sustained nourishments and different enhancements. It is generally used by the body to create new cells and nucleic destructive (which is a type of hereditary material). It is fundamental for the stable development and improvement of the infant and aides in completing explicit capacities, for example, creating red platelets, securing the youngster's ability to hear, and supporting the child's organ advancement.

Specialists suggest taking 400mcg of folic corrosive alongside pre-birth nutrients consistently previously and during pregnancy.

For what reason Should You Take Folic Acid When Pregnant?

Here is the reason you have to expand your admission of folic corrosive if you are pregnant or are attempting to get pregnant.

1. Avoids neural cylinder absconds:

Folic corrosive aides in the neural improvement of the hatchling. The neural container of your hatchling, which later develops into the mind and spinal rope of your child, is secured by folic corrosive to anticipate any pre-birth deserts during the new arrangement of the focal sensory system.

2. Produces red platelets:

Folate upgrades the generation of red platelets in your body. This is indispensable during pregnancy when weakness (iron inadequacy) is a typical protest. Folic corrosive guarantees that the red platelet (RBC) include in your body is standard in any event when you take different enhancements that could recharge the iron.

3. Shields the infant from a few confusions:

Folic corrosive brings down the infant's danger of congenital fissure and a sense of taste. It additionally lessens the risk of untimely birth, unproductive labour, and poor child development in your belly and low birth weight issues.

4. Ensures hopeful mom:

Sufficient admission of folic corrosive consistently is known to forestall preeclampsia, heart stroke, coronary illness, tumors, and Alzheimer's infection.

5. Other fundamental capacities:

Folic corrosive is required for the generation, fix, and working of DNA. It is likewise significant for the speedy development of the placenta and creating infant.

Given its significance, folic corrosive should be taken even before you get pregnant.

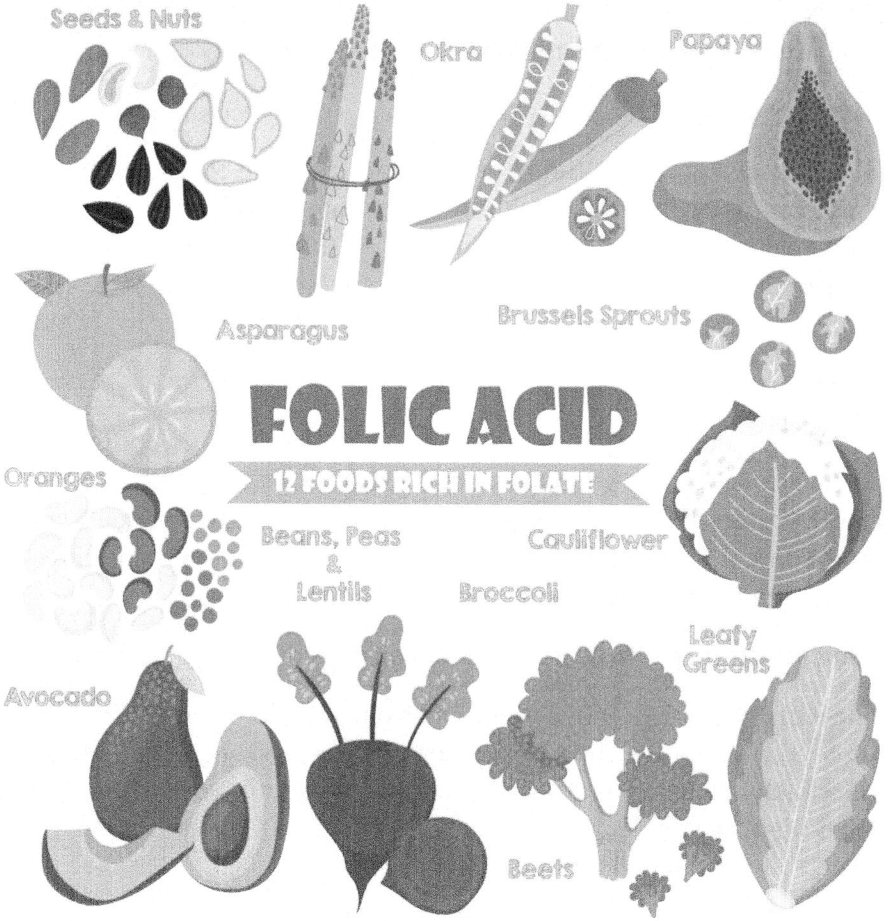

When Should You Start Taking Folic Acid?

Your PCP will encourage you to begin taking folic corrosive when you intend to consider it. Taking into account that most birth deformities could create in the first trimester, expending folate even before you imagine can be amazingly useful.

Counsel your social insurance supplier before picking your pre-birth nutrients and ensure that it has the suggested measures of folate you need.

The amount Folic Acid Do You Need?

The standard separation of prescribed folic corrosive utilization previously, after and during pregnancy is as per the following:

• Before imagining: 400mcg

• The first trimester of pregnancy: 400mcg

• Second and third trimesters of pregnancy: 600mcg

• Breastfeeding stage: 500mcg

Counsel your primary care physician to see how much folic corrosive you need to devour, considering different enhancements you are taking and nutrient inadequacies on the off chance that you have any.

To what extent Do You Need To Take Folic Acid During Pregnancy?

You can begin taking folic corrosive at any rate three months before pregnancy and all through the pregnancy to bring down the danger of birth absconds.

What Are The Effects Of Folic Acid Deficiency During Pregnancy?

Inadequacy of folic corrosive will prompt pregnancy weakness with indications, for example, diminished craving, fair skin, absence of vitality, loose bowels, cerebral pain, and crabbiness. On account of a moderate insufficiency, you may not encounter any side effects yet will come up short on the fundamental measure of folate required for a child's early stage improvement.

Folic Acid Food Sources

Folate is found in a few nourishments however is water-dissolvable and effectively annihilated or dispensed with when cooked. In this way, the ideal path is to cook them only a smidgen or eat crude if conceivable. Steaming or boiling by microwave is additionally excellent.

Here is a rundown of nourishments rich in folic corrosive. Folate per half cup of serving:

• Cooked spinach: 131mcg

• Fortified breakfast grains: 100mcg

- Black-looked at peas: 101mcg
- Asparagus: 89mcg
- White rice: 90mcg
- Brussels grows 78mcg.
- Spaghetti: 83mcg
- Romaine lettuce: 64mcg
- Avocado: 59mcg
- Raw spinach: 58mcg

Some other great wellsprings of folate are cabbage, green beans, mushrooms, sweet corn, zucchini, grapefruit, orange, vegetables, squeezes, nuts, and eggs.

When Should You Stop Taking Folic Acid?

You can quit taking folic corrosive once you arrive at 12 weeks of pregnancy since the child's spine will be all around created by at that point. Notwithstanding, you can keep taking folate post the twelfth week, as it won't hurt you or your child in any capacity.

Which folic acid tablets are great to take previously or during pregnancy?

Probably the most regularly utilized folic corrosive enhancements are from the brands, for example, Nature's Blend, Now Foods and Nature's Bounty.

How does folic corrosive assistance when you are attempting to get pregnant?

Folic corrosive can improve your odds of getting pregnant, as it supports fruitfulness and promotes RBC generation other than giving other medical advantages.

Are folic corrosive and pre-birth nutrients the equivalent?

Folic corrosive is as of now present in the pre-birth nutrient recipes. If there is any requirement for additional folate, your PCP may endorse extra folic corrosive enhancements.

What amount of folic corrosive is required for the pregnancy of twins?

Ladies conveying twins need about 1000mcg of folate every day.

Could folic corrosive admission during pregnancy cause looseness of the bowels?

Folic corrosive lack can cause the runs. In such a case, try to drink enough water to keep away from lack of hydration and look for the specialist's assistance to control the looseness of the bowels.

Will folic acid reason different pregnancies?

No, acid, folic supplementation before pregnancy won't improve the probability of numerous pregnancies.

Is an excessive amount of folic corrosive awful for pregnancy?

Indeed, an excessive amount of folic corrosive can build your infant's danger of creating mental imbalance, weight, insulin opposition, and subjective impedance.

Folic corrosive is necessary to get pregnant and for the improvement of the embryo during pregnancy; however, alert ought to be taken to maintain a strategic distance from unreasonable admission of the nutrient. Likewise, beyond what many would consider possible, attempt to get the nutrient from usual nourishment sources and use supplements just whenever recommended by the specialist. Converse with your obstetrician or nutritionist to devise a perfect diet intend to enhance your body with adequate supplements.

Itching Belly During Pregnancy

Envision scratching your belly constantly. Regardless of whether you are at home, at work, in a gathering, or a forum, one hand is occupied continuously at it on your stomach. It could appear to be strange to the spectators, yet just a pregnant lady can see that it is so hard to control the desire to scratch an itching belly during pregnancy. While you may get brief help when you scratch, the central issue is on the off chance that you should scratch or not scratch.

Is It Normal To Have An Itchy Belly During Pregnancy?

Indeed, it is very typical for the developing belly to be bothersome because of the extending skin. Sometimes, your breasts, palms, and soles turn bothersome as well. This is because of the hormonal changes and skin conditions that create with advancing pregnancy. On the off chance that the itching quits fooling around, you ought to quickly counsel your social insurance professional.

When Can You Have Itching Around The Belly Area?

An irritated belly, for the most part, happens in the second trimester, i.e., somewhere in the range of 13 and 28 weeks. However, it could happen in the first or third trimester also. Itching is increasingly conspicuous in the event of twin pregnancy, as the skin may extend more than it does in a healthy pregnancy.

What Causes The Belly To Itch During Pregnancy?

Mild itching is normal and isn't a worry. It's for the most part occurs because of reasons:

Extending belly: Most regularly, irritated stomach creates because of the developing uterus. The skin stretches and extends, becomes dampness denied, dries out, and feels angry. Treating the dryness would take care of the issue.

Hormonal floods: Hormonal changes, particularly the expansion in estrogen levels are another reason for the itching sensation on the stomach.

Is Itching During Pregnancy Dangerous?

Sometimes, a bothersome belly can be an indication of a genuine ailment. Alongside extreme itching, rashes may create.

1. Pruritic urticarial papules and plaques of pregnancy (PUPPS):

• PUPPS is a condition portrayed by bothersome red knocks on the pregnant belly and large patches of the hive-like rashes.

• Nearly 1% of pregnant ladies build up this condition, which is likewise called polymorphic ejection of pregnancy.

• They could happen in the third trimester or the most recent five weeks of pregnancy, and sometimes show up after delivery.

• The reason for PUPPS is obscure, and ladies conveying twins or more, and those conveying their first child are progressively helpless to it.

• Sometimes, PUPPS can spread out to different pieces of your body, for example, thighs, bum, back, arms, and legs. They could once in a while spread to your face, neck, and hands.

• Your specialist will ordinarily endorse a topical balm.

• If the force of the condition is high, antihistamine or oral steroids are prescribed.

• PUPPS is innocuous to the unborn infant and vanishes after delivery.

• It once in a while happens in progressive pregnancies.

2. Prurigo and pregnancy:

• If you notice light emissions that start as bug nibbles (and change into cuts as you scratch), you might be experiencing a severe bothersome condition called prurigo.

• It is otherwise called well-known emissions of pregnancy, happening on stomach, appendages or middle, and create in the late second or early third trimesters.

• Treatment incorporates topical salves and antihistamines as in PUPPS, and oral steroids in severe cases.

• Prurigo is innocuous to your child and vanishes not long after delivery. Now and again, it could keep awake to a quarter of a year post-delivery.

• They can happen in progressive pregnancies.

3. Pemphigoid gestationis:

• Pemphigoid gestationis is an excellent skin condition where irritated ejections start as hives and transform into enormous, estimated rankles or sores.

• It is otherwise called herpes gestationis because of its infection like appearance.

• These in all likelihood show up in the second or third trimesters, and even one to about fourteen days after delivery.

• It begins close to the belly catch and spreads to the storage compartment, arms, legs, palms, and soles. Oral steroids are recommended for treatment. Pemphigoid gestationis that erupts after delivery is said to decrease with breastfeeding.

• This condition is more genuine than PUPPS and is known to trigger pre-term labour, fetal development issues, and even stillbirth. This implies you should check with a specialist when you see the signs.

• In uncommon cases, an infant may build up a rash that is generally mellow and dies down in half a month. This condition can happen in progressive pregnancies and could be more severe than in the prior pregnancy.

4. Impetigo herpetiformis:

• Impetigo herpetiformis isn't brought about by herpes infection, yet it is a skin disease and a type of psoriasis in pregnancy.

• It creates in the third trimester and is described by red patches loaded up with discharge that gradually develop into more significant discharge filled white rashes.

• These patches may show up on your thighs, crotch, belly, armpits, under the breasts, and other areas. Impetigo herpetiformis is related to queasiness, regurgitating, the runs, fever, and chills.

• This condition is treated with foundational corticosteroids, and you will be under perception.

• It vanishes after delivery and can repeat in the progressive pregnancies.

5. Intrahepatic cholestasis of pregnancy (ICP):

• ICP is a severe condition that triggers tremendous itching. This is an uncommon condition, and about 1% of pregnancy cases in the US have announced it.

• It creates in the third trimester and is a condition associated with the liver where bile doesn't stream regularly. Instead, bile salts aggregate in the skin, causing severe tingle, rashes, and hives.

• You are probably going to create red rashes for the most part on soles, palms, and stomach. Side effects of ICP incorporate sickness, discomfort, and loss of craving.

• ICP is amazingly dangerous and can prompt stillbirth.

These conditions have comparable signs. At the point when you notice any skin issues, you should check with your primary care physician, who will perceive the precise problem and treat you as needs be.

When To Consult A Doctor?

Call your social insurance supplier on the off chance that you:

• Develop extreme tingle on the stomach and other body parts.

• Experience any tingle not identified with dry or touchy skin.

• The tingle spreads everywhere throughout the body.

• Have severe itching and rashes, which could be expected to PUPP or ICP, in the third trimester.

• Develop itching joined by light shaded solid discharges, dark-hued pee, spewing, queasiness, weariness, and loss of craving.

If the itching isn't related to any wellbeing condition, at that point, necessary home cures or over-the-counter arrangements can give alleviation.

Home Remedies For Itchy Belly During Pregnancy:

Here are some protected and common cures that you can go after itching, rashes, pain, and expanding.

1. Oats shower for irritated skin:

Add some cereal to warm water and wash with it. It calms the troubled skin and decreases irritation. You could likewise tie knee-high nylon socks, loaded up with steel cut cereal, to the tap. At the point when you utilize the warm faucet water that has gone through those socks, it will give alleviation and help you unwind.

2. Preparing soft drink shower:

Pour half cup of making the soft drink in warm water, and absorb it for whatever length of time that you get help. Lean toward heating soft drink to developing the powder as the soft drink is progressively successful in soothing the tingle and skin irritation. You can likewise make a glue of preparing pop and water and apply on the belly and other bothersome regions.

3. Aloe vera gel:

Use aloe vera gel to every one of those bothersome and disturbing skin regions not long after a shower. It will mitigate and diminish aggravation. The aloe vera gel layer will shield the skin and keep from any harm when you will, in general, scratch on the stomach.

4. Cold pack:

Apply a virus pack on your belly with wool or washcloth absorbed virus water to lessen the irritating sensation. You can likewise utilize it notwithstanding cereal or preparing soft drink shower.

5. Saturate:

Touch a little cream that is delicate and aroma free. Applying this often will incidentally alleviate the itching.

6. Coconut oil:

Apply the oil on the irritated belly all through your pregnancy to moderate dryness and irritation.

7. Apple juice vinegar:

You can put some apple juice vinegar on the bothersome stomach as it works superbly in soothing aggravation and dryness.

Over-The-Counter Products For Itchy Belly:

1. Oil-based lotions:

The items are perfect for a bothersome belly as they are effectively retained into your skin. You can get them at any excellence path or medication store. On the off chance that you need to include aroma, put a couple of drops of fundamental oils, for example, lavender or frankincense into the cream. The quieting aroma will die down any expanding.

Some fundamental oils, for example, nutmeg, rosemary, jasmine, basil, rose, clary sage, and juniper, are not suggested during pregnancy.

2. Calamine moisturizer:

Apply limited quantities of calamine on the irritated stomach a few times in a day. Calamine contains zinc carbonate, zinc, and iron oxides, which help diminish irritated skin.

3. Nutrient E salve:

You can forestall itching during pregnancy by applying nutrient E cream or container oil, accessible at nearby medication stores. Use nutrient E with some restraint as high sums may expand the danger of heart issues in the infant.

Notwithstanding the home and OTC cures, you may play it safe to control the spread of the sensation.

Step by step instructions to Prevent Itchy Belly During Pregnancy:

While you can fail to address the beginning of itching, you can take gauges either to diminish or keep the irritation from exasperating. Embrace the accompanying advances:

• Avoid high temp water shower or showers as they can trigger irritation. Instead, utilize warm water for washing.

• Do not utilize solid smelling cleansers and gels as they lead to dry skin. Utilize soft shampoo or shower gels that are delicate on the surface.

• Wear-free attire that is perfect and dry. Tight and wet garments will rub against the skin, influencing the dryness and irritating.

• Do not remain in the sun or sweltering climate as they can dry the skin, prompting irritation. Likewise, the UV beams from the sun are known to bother the rashes on the dry skin.

• Moisturize your skin now and again and enough. Utilize great lotions that have an unbiased pH.

• Avoid being in the AC for extensive stretches as that also can dry your skin and lead to irritation and bothering.

• Drink enough water (around eight to ten glasses per day) as it hydrates your body and saturates your skin regularly.

The reasons for a bothersome belly during pregnancy are shifted. Try not to disregard any tingle or rash. Converse with your primary care physician, and on the off chance that she says it is not something to be stressed over, at that point, you may utilize some OTC creams or home solutions for itching during pregnancy that the specialist suggests.

Sixth Month Pregnancy Diet - Which Foods To Eat And Avoid?

The sixth month implies you are in charge of the sickness, and your food cravings might be expanding, as the child needs more nutrition to develop at this stage. Needing to eat continually is a typical piece of the sixth month during your pregnancy. Notwithstanding eating routinely, you additionally need to eat right, as all that you eat now will assume an enormous job in your infant's improvement. This is the reason you must incorporate sound nourishments sixth month of pregnancy diet to be fit as a fiddle for the birth, just as give the perfect measure of nutrition for your unborn youngster.

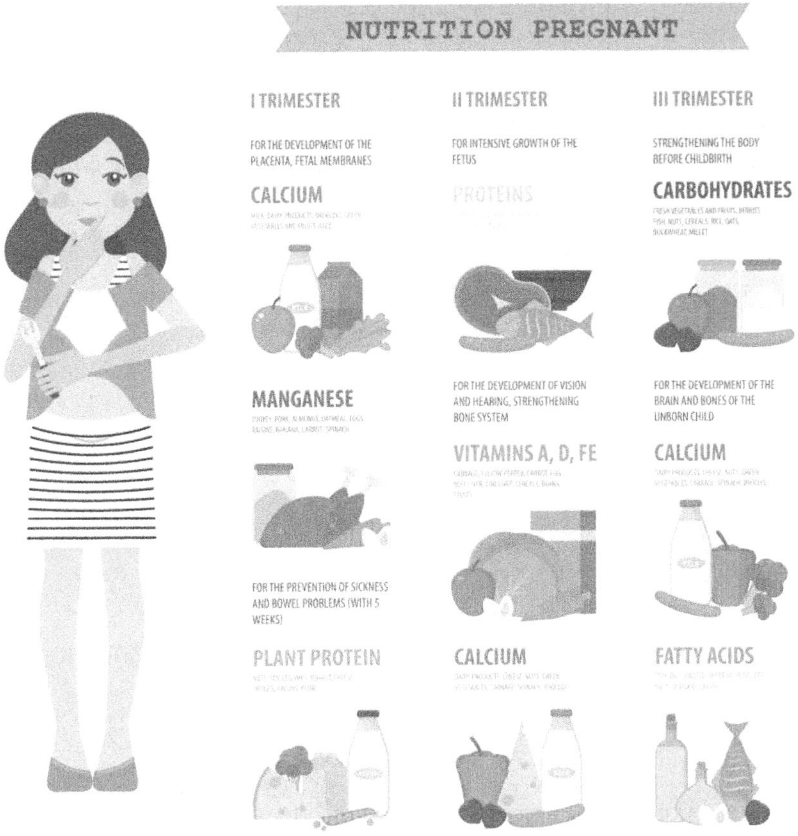
NUTRITION PREGNANT
I TRIMESTER
II TRIMESTER
III TRIMESTER
FOR THE DEVELOPMENT OF THE PLACENTA, FETAL MEMBRANES
CALCIUM
FOR INTENSIVE GROWTH OF THE FETUS
PROTEINS
STRENGTHENING THE BODY BEFORE CHILDBIRTH
CARBOHYDRATES
MANGANESE
FOR THE DEVELOPMENT OF VISION AND HEARING, STRENGTHENING BONE SYSTEM
VITAMINS A, D, FE
FOR THE DEVELOPMENT OF THE BRAIN AND BONES OF THE UNBORN CHILD
CALCIUM
FOR THE PREVENTION OF SICKNESS AND BOWEL PROBLEMS (WITH 5 WEEKS)
PLANT PROTEIN
CALCIUM
FATTY ACIDS

Diet For Sixth Month Of Pregnancy?

Eating well is of most extreme significance all through your pregnancy, particularly since your child is developing quickly. All that you eat will add to your infant's improvement and development, so you have to give additional consideration towards your day by day diet. Before you pursue the beneath referenced diet, recall that each lady's body is unique, and what might be useful for others may not function admirably for you. Make sure to check the diet with your primary care physician before you start any of the things referenced. Additionally, avoid whatever your wellbeing consultant may have requested that you stay away from.

Here are a few nourishments that you should make a piece of your diet during the sixth month of pregnancy:

1. Protein:

This significant supplement ought to be a piece of your day by day diet. In any case, you ought to evade greasy fish and the skin, additionally meat fat. It is, in certainty, a smart thought to maintain a strategic distance from an excessive amount of meat, and particularly red meat.

You ought to go for:

• Lean meat

• Whitefish

• Eggs

• Black beans

• Tofu

These nourishments will profit you and your kid by giving you the protein that your body requires.

2. Sugars:

A bit or two per day of sugars is suggested during pregnancy. However, remember this relies upon how a lot of weight you have picked up.

You ought to go for:

• Potatoes

• Pasta

• Sweet corn

• Seeds and nuts

• Oats

These are a portion of the nourishments that are rich in 'carbs' and sound as well.

3. Vegetables:

The decency of vegetables is no mystery, and during your sixth month of pregnancy, they are a much increasingly significant piece of your diet.

You ought to go for:

• Beetroot

• Cabbage

• Asparagus

• Spinach

• Carrots

• Pumpkin

• Turnip

• Eggplant/Brinjal

• Green beans

• Tomatoes

These tasty vegetables will do a ton of good for your child and you.

4. Organic products:

There is not at all like fresh, natural products to revive and renew you. The decency that they pack in makes them the best nourishment to eat while you are pregnant.

You ought to go for:

• Bananas

• Grapes

• Kiwis

• Apples

• Pears

• Clementine

• Oranges

These are extraordinary wellsprings of supplements that will help in your infant's advancement and development, so load up on these tasty nourishments!

5. Dairy Products:

If you maintained a strategic distance from dairy items before your pregnancy, presently is the ideal time to enjoy! The calcium you take in will help in ensuring that your infant's bones become solid. If you are stressed over putting on overabundance weight, you can settle on skimmed or low-fat dairy items. You don't have to stress as these areas yet wealthy in calcium just as protein. Nonetheless, ensure you check with your PCP, as certain ladies create lactose prejudice during this stage, while a few specialists may request that you remain off skimmed milk.

You ought to go for:

- Yogurt
- Cheese
- Milk

6. Liquids:

You should drink a lot of water and natural product juices during this phase of your pregnancy. Specialists prescribe 6 to 8 glasses of fluids consistently to renew your body and give your infant essential minerals that are available in the water. Crisp natural product juices will provide you with the vital supplements to have a healthy pregnancy and child!

Diet To Avoid In The Sixth Month Of Pregnancy

Numerous ladies regularly have longings for rather unfortunate nourishments while they are pregnant. While it is alright to enjoy tolerably in some low-quality nourishment, there are sure food sources that ought to be kept away from while you are pregnant, particularly up to your sixth month.

Here is a portion of the nourishments that are flat out no-no during your pregnancy:

1. Crude Seafood:

You may have a sudden craving for sushi yet maintain a strategic distance from it no matter what! As coarse fish convey a significant level of methyl mercury that can cause nourishment borne illnesses like listeriosis, which can be unsafe for your unborn child.

2. Half-cooked Meat:

Continuously ensure that you cook your meat well as the microbes referenced above can be available in half-cooked beef. On the off chance that you are preparing meat for supper, take care to cook it well with the goal that you can process it effectively and keep away from the danger of listeriosis. Attempt to abstain from eating meat outside.

3. Non-Pasteurized Cheeses:

Maintain a strategic distance from delicate cheeses that are not purified and stick to hard cheeses just during your pregnancy, particularly during your sixth month. Malady causing microbes can likewise be available in this sort of cheddar, so preclude it from your diet.

4. Fiery Food:

There will be times when you need to eat something hot and passionate; notwithstanding, it is ideal to abstain from whatever is excessively zesty. It can make your stomach copy and cause acid reflux and extraordinary distress. It is additionally not probably the best flavor to give your child, so check your desires for anything excessively zesty.

5. Caffeine:

It is ideal for maintaining a strategic distance from juiced refreshments, for example, espresso and circulated air through beverages. It is a lot more beneficial choice to drink natural tea as it will soothe and quiet you, which is actually what you need while you are pregnant. On the other hand, check with your primary care physician, as certain ladies are put off green or natural tea during pregnancy.

6. Liquor And Tobacco:

It's an undeniable fact that you have to avoid alcohol and tobacco while you are pregnant totally. The harm done to your child can be unsalvageable, even deadly, when you smoke or drink during pregnancy.

Keep in mind:

Aside from these nourishments, you ought to likewise abstain from taking any over the counter medicine. If you have a condition that expects you to take medication, counsel your primary care physician and see whether it is sheltered to be taken while you are pregnant. Just the meds and enhancements endorsed by your primary care physician ought to be taken, and it is of most extreme significance to see whether some other meds you are taking are alright for your child. Ensure you make it exceptionally obvious to the primary care physician that you are pregnant.

Eating a decent diet and furnishing your body and your child with all the necessary supplements required ought to be your essential objective. At the point when you ensure that what you take in regularly is sound and gainful for your child's improvement and development, you guarantee that your infant grows up to be skipping, stable little holy messenger!

Remain solid and deal with yourself just as your child. A solid mother conveys a sound child, so recall your wellbeing is of most extreme significance as well!

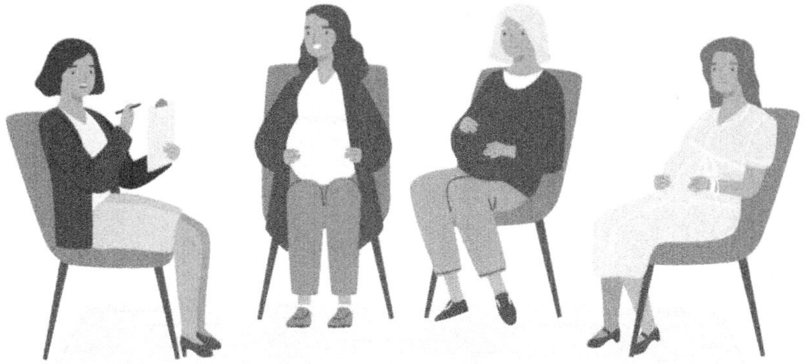

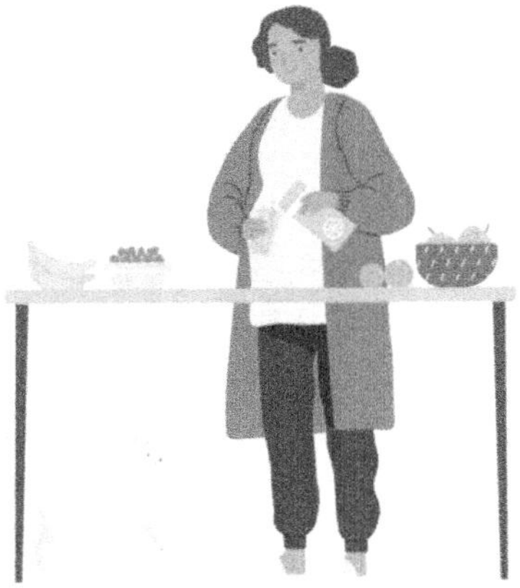

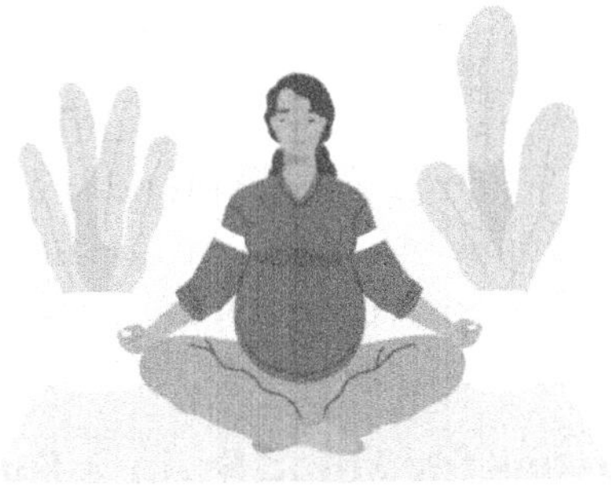

"The moment a child is born, the mother is also born. She never existed before. The woman existed, but the mother, never. A mother is something absolutely new." and so in you the child your mother lives on and through your family continues to live... so at this time look after yourself and your family as you would your mother" - *Osho*

CHAPTER FOUR

PREGNANCY SECRETS THAT NO ONE EVER TELLS YOU ABOUT

Mood Swings During Pregnancy: Causes And Management

Do you feel cheerful for quite a while and on edge and discouraged later? Do you get irritable and irritated for unimportant things or no explanation? On the off chance that you are pregnant and have responded to yes to these inquiries, stress not. Mood swings are normal during pregnancy, attributable to the hormonal, physical, and enthusiastic changes occurring inside you. While you can't evade them, you can manage them to make your pregnancy less distressing.

Reasons for Mood Swings During Pregnancy

A ton of changes occurring in the body, both physically and rationally could be liable for mood swings all through the pregnancy.

1. Hormonal variance maybe the regular reason for mood changes. At the point when you get pregnant, the degree of pregnancy hormones (progesterone and estrogen) increments. This usually brings about sentiments of nervousness, pity, dread, and dissatisfaction which can prompt sadness.

2. Extreme tiredness and morning disorder are commonly experienced during the first and second trimesters. These could be liable for changes in your mood. You may have a blend of feelings, for example, neglect, moodiness, and even nervousness.

3. Lack of rest because of the developing belly and other pregnancy changes is another reason for mood swings. Inadequate rest can make you feel bothered and irritable.

4. Health conditions, for example, hypothyroidism, gestational diabetes, and paleness, could be liable for mood swings too. They are connected to sentiments of wretchedness, dread, bothering, and exhaustion during pregnancy.

Independent of the causes behind them, mood swings are sensible.

How To Deal With Mood Swings During Pregnancy?

A solid diet, joined with a couple of way of life changes, could assist you with unwinding and deal with your mood better.

1. Indulge in reflection and yoga: Most pregnant ladies experience sentiments of nervousness, wretchedness, and trouble. As indicated by an investigation, yoga and contemplation work on during pregnancy can help lessen the side effects of gloom.

2. Get legitimate rest: Lack of rest is one of the regular reasons for mood swings. Attempt to limit rest unsettling influences by making an agreeable rest schedule: wear-free/pleasing garments, diminish the lights in your room, abstain from utilizing contraptions before rest, and use cushions for help.

3. Get a pre-birth knead: A pre-birth back rub can assuage your muscles and lessen pain and help in the working of the lymphatic and circulatory frameworks, in this way improving your mood and helping you remain quiet.

4. Pamper yourself: You can attempt necessary, yet fun exercises like shopping, eating something that you are longing for, taking a stroll with your accomplice, viewing a motion picture, or investing some quality energy with your friends and family. Anything that makes you feel better works.

5. Talk to your accomplice: Sometimes, quietly conversing with your accomplice about your emotions can enable you to unwind. Vent out when you have to and don't pressure yourself by overthinking about everything.

6. Stay aware of different pregnancy-related perspectives: You may have a ton of fears about pregnancy and labor. Some could be substantial, yet most could be nonsensical because of the absence of information. So

converse with your primary care physician and clear any questions you have about the pregnancy, diet, tests, pre-birth care, or wellbeing conditions, and settle on the correct choices.

7. Stay solid: Health conditions (gestational diabetes, hyperthyroidism, or paleness) could make you worried too. Try not to disregard them or overthink them – instead, center on overseeing them by taking meds and following the recommendations of your primary care physician.

It's Okay To Have Mood Swings

Realize that it's alright to feel whatever you feel during pregnancy. Try not to battle it or harp on it. Acknowledge how you think and pursue the tips to deal with your moods for better mental and physiological wellbeing. Realizing that your sentiments can be overseen can lessen pressure radically. You should make little way of life changes and discover more approaches to feel much improved and appreciate the pregnancy.

Worry During Pregnancy: Its Signs, Effects, And Tips To Reduce It

Stress and uneasiness about pregnancy and labor are normal in pregnant ladies. A tad of nervousness, dissatisfaction, and melancholy are okay and nothing to be stressed over. In any case, on the off chance that you will, in general, stress excessively and experience alarm more than you'd need to, it is a reason for concern.

What Causes Stress During Pregnancy?

The reasons for pressure vary from lady to lady. For certain moms, to-be, being pregnant is distressing in itself. They think that it's challenging to remain in charge and deal with the physical changes.

Different reasons that could negatively affect a to-be mom include:

• Experiencing physical worry because of pregnancy indications, for example, queasiness, obstruction, laziness or body hurts, and managing them.

• Hormonal vacillations prompting mood swings could influence mental constitution, making it harder to deal with pressure.

• Managing occupation, pregnancy, and family tasks could be hard for a few. It may influence their own and expert life and could add to the pressure.

• Domestic misuse and other individual issues could likewise cause pressure other than having hurtful results.

If you are encountering more than one of the above circumstances throughout your life, your feelings of anxiety could be a lot higher.

What Types Of Stress Can Cause Pregnancy Problems?

Stress can be dealt with as long as you most likely are aware of overseeing it without exasperating it. Regular pressure, for example, coping with cutoff times and driving in rush hour gridlock, may not add to the current pregnancy issues. In any case, different kinds of stress can cause devastation during pregnancy.

• Negative educational encounters, for example, a bombed marriage and separation, deadly illnesses, the passing of a friend or family member, or losing a vocation can cause extreme pressure that is difficult to deal with.

• Unfortunate occasions, including ordinary catastrophes, for example, tropical storms, tremors, floods, or human-made debacles, for instance, psychological militant assaults or mishaps may make a profound, passionate effect during pregnancy, prompting mental pressure.

• Acute worry because of monetary issues, relationship issues, physical or mental maltreatment could influence you the most noticeably awful, and may likewise prompt long-haul despondency.

• Some ladies are probably going to encounter worry from the supremacist comments or assaults. This is one reason why African-American ladies in the US bring forth low birth weight and untimely infants.

• Pregnancy stress that stems from fears of the unnatural birth cycle, labor pain, child's wellbeing, or nerves of turning into a parent is one more reason for worry in ladies. This could make one restless, hyper, and even discouraged.

How Does Stress Affect Your Pregnancy?

Stress is probably not going to cause severe results on the off chance that it is overseen appropriately. It could influence the strength of both the mother-to-be and the child at times. Extreme, prolonged haul pressure can cause the accompanying intricacies when left untreated:

• High circulatory strain

• Gestational diabetes

• Weakened safe framework

• Severe wretchedness

A few ladies attempt to oversee worry by smoking, liquor utilization, and admission of medications, which could again prompt genuine medical issues in the mother and the child.

By what method Can Stress Affect Your Unborn Baby?

Worry during pregnancy can influence the unborn from multiple points of view.

• Emotional stress animates the arrival of cortisol hormone, which increments with the seriousness of importance. This could cause wretchedness, weight, muscle misfortune, heart ailment, and osteoporosis in the infant sometime down the road.

• The infant is probably going to conceived preterm, which could bring about stomach related issues, respiratory issues, low insusceptibility, and passing of the baby now and again.

• Even full-term children might be brought into the world underweight and have shortcoming and inadequate safe framework. It can likewise cause hypoxia (insufficient oxygen supply during the birth time), which can prompt long-haul formative results in babies.

• Increased danger of Attention Deficit Hyperactivity Disorder (ADHD) in later life.

What Are The Symptoms Of Stress During Pregnancy?

Incessant pressure can cause numerous physical, passionate, mental, and social manifestations including.

• Chest pain, breathing challenges, vision issues, migraines, quick heartbeat, discombobulation, exhaustion, muscle throbs, stomach issues, and expanded perspiring.

• Confusion, bad dreams, memory misfortune, changes in the sleeping example, and trouble centering.

• Grief, blame, uneasiness, fractiousness, dread, forswearing, stress, depression, or disappointment

• Isolation from loved ones, eating less, medication, and liquor misuse.

Approaches To Manage Stress During Pregnancy

Stress is anything but complicated to oversee when you remember it accurately and realize how to deal with it. It will prompt a positive pregnancy encounter and diminish the danger of wellbeing complexities for you and your child.

Here are a few different ways to decrease worry during pregnancy.

• Indulge in some light physical activity, for example, strolling as it brings down feelings of anxiety as well as forestalls regular pregnancy inconveniences.

• Try unwinding procedures, for example, pre-birth yoga or contemplation.

• Learn to do breathing exercises.

• Just relax and loosen up at whatever point conceivable.

• Get engaged with exercises, for example, perusing a book, viewing your preferred show, or doing a few activities you appreciate.

• Figure out what is focusing on you more, and have a go at discussing it with your accomplice, a companion, or even an advisor if necessary.

• Seek support from loved ones – request that they take you to pre-birth tests or help you with the family errands.

• Go for labor instruction classes to comprehend about pregnancy, labor, unwinding strategies, and exercises.

• Get ventures at work done before and abstain from delaying them to the last moment to keep worried under control.

• If you think you are discouraged, go to treatment right off the bat to keep away from the requirement for antidepressants.

• Eat sound and nutritious nourishment.

• Consider joining a care group to meet similarly invested pregnant ladies.

Become familiar with stress and pregnancy next, where we address some usually raised questions.

Will pressure influence early pregnancy?

Worry during the first trimester is known to influence the microbial populace in the mother's vagina. These can be passed onto babies during birth, in this way causing an effect on the digestion and resistant arrangement of the newborn child. Modified gut microflora is additionally known to expand the danger of neurodevelopmental issues, for example, schizophrenia and chemical imbalance.

Would you be able to have an unnatural birth cycle because of stress?

No, contemplates don't show that pressure can cause premature delivery. Notwithstanding, extreme stress can prompt untimely birth, low birth weight, or conduct issues sometime down the road.

Will pressure influence pregnancy in the third trimester?

Extreme worry during the third trimester will raise maternal cortisol levels, which can lastingly affect a kid's psychological capacities and IQ scores.

Does pressure cause birth deserts?

Serious worry during pregnancy is probably going to cause birth imperfections, for example, congenital fissure, spina bifida, anencephaly, and natural heart deserts.

Will crying influence pregnancy?

Crying during pregnancy is because of passionate pressure and sorrow. It is related to preterm labour, lower birth weight babies, and intrauterine development limitations.

Being focused on is unpleasant, yet recall that you are not the only one. There is help on the off chance that you request it. You may suddenly encounter pressure. However, all you have to know is how to oversee it well. If you can't adapt to pressure, converse with your PCP about what is causing you stress, and get arrangements.

Cryptic Pregnancy: Causes, Signs And Duration

What Is A Cryptic Pregnancy?

A cryptic pregnancy is one that goes undetected or unnoticed until delivery. It alludes to a restoratively characterized condition called 'refusal of pregnancy.' This implies you are pregnant. However, the human chorionic gonadotropin (hCG) levels are too low to be distinguished in a blood or pee test, possibly.

Cryptic pregnancies, for the most part, happen in ladies who have been on anti-conception medication strategies, for example, contraceptive pills, IUCD, tubal ligation (tubes attached to keep the sperm from entering the fallopian tunnel), and so on. These ladies go under the 'least anticipated pregnancy classification' and experience regular pregnancy manifestations, for example, exhaustion and morning infection gently, or don't encounter anything by any means. These manifestations are mixed up as those of some other condition.

What Causes Cryptic Pregnancy?

A few hormonal and mental reasons can prompt cryptic pregnancy. In any case, the psychological causes are lower than the hormonal.

1. Polycystic ovarian disorder (PCOS): Small sores structure on the broadened ovaries. Ladies may have irregular or drawn-out cycles because of hormonal irregularity.

2. Recent pregnancy: Hormones may return time to get to typical after your pregnancy. Ongoing labor and lactation may cause amenorrhea, and ladies probably won't know when they began ovulating once more. On the off chance that you are pregnant quickly, there would be hormonal irregularity causing a cryptic pregnancy.

3. Low body fat could trigger a hormonal lopsidedness as on account of competitors.

4. Perimenopause is the time when the body fires, giving up indications of movement to menopause, prompting irregular cycles. It can begin as right on time as during the 30's, causing the pregnancy to go unidentified.

5. Birth control pills, for example, Deprovera, Norplant, or Mirena Coil, discharge more hormones that influence the ordinary pregnancy hormones making them helpless against pregnancy.

6. High-feelings of anxiety can cause a cryptic pregnancy as they impact the hormones.

What Is The Duration Of Cryptic Pregnancy?

There is no proof to decide the length or the growth time of cryptic pregnancy. That is fundamental because the lady probably won't know when the pregnancy began, to what extent it might go, and when it would end. Notwithstanding, it is said that a cryptic pregnancy endures more extended than the normal pregnancy as the improvement is slower. In any case, this did not depend on any exploration or study.

Sometimes, there could be regular periods during a cryptic pregnancy because of incomplete shedding of the endometrial coating. Indeed, even in such a case, it gets hard to decide the length. Some enigmatic pregnancy cases that have been accounted for were shorter than typical pregnancy, while some were longer. Consequently, the range is unsure. In any event, when the pregnancy is cryptic, it could send you a few signs.

MY BAD SYMPTOMS DURING PREGNANCY

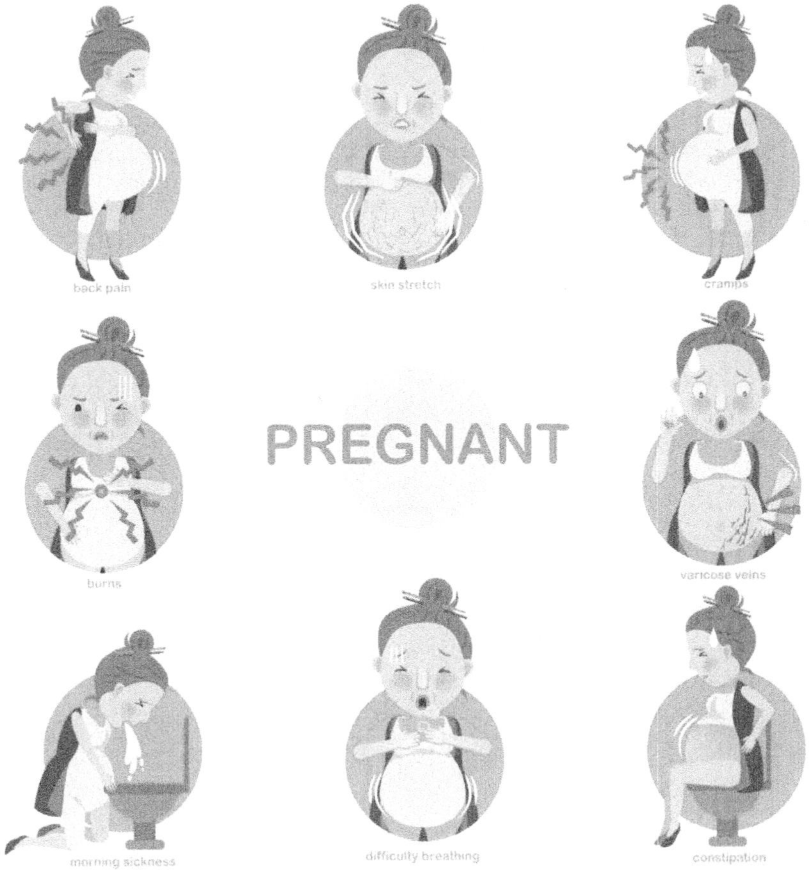
back pain
skin stretch
cramps
PREGNANT
burns
varicose veins
morning sickness
difficulty breathing
constipation

Do you encounter any of the symptoms in the image? Which?

Bleeding? ______________________________

____

Abundant salivation? ______________________________

____

Insomnia or anxiety? ______________________________

____

Itch? ______________________________

____

Hemorrhoids? ______________________________

Severe complications? ______________________________

____

____

Cryptic Pregnancy Symptoms

The side effects of cryptic pregnancy are like a healthy pregnancy. Note that the side effects differ from one lady to the next.

- Nausea
- Vomiting
- Fatigue
- Food repugnance
- Frequent pee
- Weight gain
- Heartburn
- Headaches
- Abdominal cramps
- Backache
- Metallic taste in the mouth

The manifestations could be like those of a healthy pregnancy. Things being what they are, how is cryptic pregnancy not the same as the regular?

Why Is Cryptic Pregnancy Cryptic?

Pregnancy stays a mystery given these reasons:

- You may have regular periods all through the pregnancy because of halfway shedding of the endometrial coating. However, the number of draining days might be less. Spotting and seeping because of implantation could be confused with a standard period.
- Urine and blood tests and ultrasound show the contrary.
- Slow pregnancy belly development as a child is at the rear of the belly (at the spine).
- Fetal developments inside the belly are confused with gas and swelling.

What Befalls The Fetus In Cryptic Pregnancy?

In cryptic pregnancy, the improvement of the baby is deferred and hindered now and again, occurring at a very moderate pace. In any case, this doesn't influence the wellbeing of the baby. The mother would go to the emergency clinic just when she has severe stomach and back issues, that is, during labor.

By what method Can Pregnancy Go Undetected After Missed Periods?

Not all ladies have customary and monthly periods, and a missed period may not trouble them. Regardless of whether periods happen once in a while, spotting during pregnancy might be interpreted as menstrual dying. The unpredictable or less stream could be credited to pressure, menopause, or other medical issues.

Proceeded with Periods/Bleeding In Cryptic Pregnancy

Most ladies keep getting their regular periods all through the cryptic pregnancy, yet this doesn't demonstrate an unnatural birth cycle. It may be overwhelming, light, or spot seeping with a couple of enormous or little clumps. The draining can be brilliant red, pink, dark-colored, purple, orange, or dark. It very well may resemble an ordinary period, sporadic or irregular. The draining could sometimes keep going for quite a long time or months. However, everything it does is shed away the uterine coating — this outcome in almost no hCG.

How Is A Negative Test Result Possible?

In a typical pregnancy, the pregnancy test shows contrary on the off chance that it is taken too soon or if you neglect to adhere to the directions effectively.

Be that as it may, in a cryptic pregnancy, the outcome is negative because the degree of hCG is irrelevant. The placenta generally secretes hCG, which goes along the coating of the uterus. It develops and is appeared in the pee and blood. In cryptic pregnancy, the covering of the uterus occasionally sheds without giving hCG the extension to create and perform in tests.

Also, on the off chance that you are not foreseeing a pregnancy, you would not step through the examination.

How Does Cryptic Pregnancy Go Undetected In Ultrasound?

In a healthy pregnancy, the specialist will do a transvaginal ultrasound 12 weeks into the pregnancy. From that point onward, she will do a stomach ultrasound until the due week.

Nonetheless, in most cryptic pregnancy cases, ultrasound can't identify the developing hatchling in a more significant part of ladies. This might be because of individual variations from the norm in the stomach district or uterus.

1. Uterine retroversion: It is otherwise called tipped or tilted uterus because the uterus is slanted towards the rear of the pelvis dissimilar to a vertical situation (as in a healthy womb). This position makes it hard to see the baby in an ultrasound during early incubation. Retroversion occurs because of one of the beneath reasons:

• The uterus doesn't move to the back position during pubescence.

• The developing infant extends the tendons, repositioning the uterus from its unique spot.

• Endometriosis (endometrium becomes outside the uterus) or fibroids (non-harmful developments in the womb) can cause scarring, which will move the uterus to the first position.

2. Bicornuate uterus: It is an inborn anomaly wherein the uterus is heart-molded with two horns. A divider parts the uterus either totally or halfway. It would thus be able to influence the conceptive capacities of a lady and bring about cryptic pregnancy.

3. Abnormal scar tissue: An unusual scar tissue can occur because of stomach medical procedure, C-segment, or belly tucks, among others. This scar tissue counteracts the ultrasound waves from going into the uterus, demonstrating adverse outcomes on the output.

For what reason Does Cryptic Pregnancy Have Longer Gestational Period?

The HCG won't go into the maternal framework as in a run of the mill pregnancy. This keeps the body from creating signals fundamental for infant advancement. The hatchling will accordingly develop gradually. The infants measure littler than they ought to be at different pregnancy stages. Likewise, regular periods during cryptic pregnancy draw out the gestational period. The heavier the period dying, the more is the incubation.

Potential Complications Of Cryptic Pregnancy

There would not be pre-birth care as you don't know about your pregnancy. The delivery, in this manner turns out to be unassisted or at home.

• Prenatal inconveniences, for example, hypertension, diabetes, or blood bunch incongruence, will go undetected, putting both the mother and infant in danger.

• The mother may not maintain a strategic distance from specific propensities, for example, smoking or drinking.

Cryptic Pregnancy Labor

Much the same as cryptic pregnancy, its labor is likewise unusual. It is long and extended, and you will encounter labor like pains for a considerable length of time before you go into real work. The labor pains, which may at first appear menstrual issues, will deteriorate and hurt much more. This, combined with the pains going on for a considerable length of time, may provoke ladies to see a specialist, where the pregnancy might be affirmed. The specialist may attempt to actuate labor or play out a C-area to convey the infant.

A portion of the labor side effects in cryptic pregnancy are:

• Back pain

• Nausea

• Vomiting

• Hot flashes

- Chills
- Dizziness
- Cold sweats
- Diarrhea
- Body hurt
- Pain in the legs that transmits to the thighs
- Mood swings
- Pain in the hip and pelvic area
- Palpitations
- Swelling of the vaginal dividers because of expanded bloodstream
- Painful breasts. Sometimes, the pain can be shooting, sharp pain.
- Pressure on the cervix
- Stabbing pain in the sides, much the same as you get in the wake of running
- Tugging or pulling sensation in the stomach area which could be painful

You may encounter all or a couple of these side effects that can extend for a considerable length of time. By and large, the real procedure of cryptic pregnancy delivery is brisk and doesn't keep going long.

You may understand back pain or a snugness that emanates to the front like that of period pain. You might need to go to the loo; however, you would not have an inside. In such a case, go to a medical clinic.

How To Prevent Cryptic Pregnancy?

During the regenerative age, on the off chance that you are persistently encountering specific pain or changes in the stomach area or pelvis, you ought to promptly observe a specialist. Even though it is hard to distinguish a pregnancy, your primary care physician may make a theory about it.

On the off chance that you don't get regular periods, take rehashed pregnancy tests. You ought to address your gynecologist about unpredictable periods and gain an exhaustive analysis. You ought to likewise complete an exam if you think you have entered menopause. Cryptic pregnancy doesn't appear to be genuine, or if nothing else, we don't see such things occurring around us.

In what capacity will the cryptic pregnancy child development be?

The sentiment of fetal developments in cryptic pregnancies resembles that of gas or fractious gut disorder. At the point when you feel your entrails and abs moving, you misconstrue them to be because of worms, blisters, blockage, fibroids, or muscle fits.

To what extent does a cryptic pregnancy last?

As the infants create at a slower pace, a cryptic pregnancy can keep going for over 40 weeks.

How to affirm a cryptic pregnancy?

Since cryptic pregnancy can't be identified through blood or pee tests, or an ultrasound check, your professional may utilize a Doppler (screens fetal pulse) alongside a finger heartbeat to affirm the pregnancy. Cryptic pregnancy can place a lady in an extreme position, particularly if she is ill-equipped to take care of an infant. A lady must be rationally, inwardly, and physically arranged to carry an infant into the world and sustain it. On the off chance that you have unpredictable periods and the test outcomes generally show, converse with a gynecologist. Additionally, deal with yourself and eat beneficial to advance an ordinary and sound improvement of your child.

Fundamental Skin Problems During Pregnancy: Symptoms And Remedies

A few ladies may encounter the pregnancy shine, while a couple may have redness or rashes on the skin. Some others may feel that their skin has gotten dull. Regardless, most skin changes during pregnancy are not destructive and generally die down before the finish of the growth time frame. Nonetheless, a couple of changes may cause inconvenience yet can be overseen through treatment or way of life changes.

What Type Of Skin Problems Occur During Pregnancy?

The skin issues that pregnant ladies form can be classified into three.

1. Pre-existing skin conditions: If you, as of now have a current skin issue, it might either improve or deteriorate with pregnancy.

2. Hormone-related skin conditions: The hormonal changes happening in the body could trigger some kindhearted (gentle) skin conditions.

3. Pregnancy-explicit skin conditions: Some of the skin changes during pregnancy are because of the different physiological changes that you experience.

A few ladies may encounter a cover of the conditions referenced previously. Most skin issues can be treated with characteristic cures or by taking drugs endorsed by the specialist. For that, you ought to have the option to analyze the skin issue precisely.

Skin Changes During Pregnancy

While some skin changes are healthy and might vanish after delivery, a couple may require treatment considerably after birth.

1. Skin inflammation

Hormonal changes, oil generation, and expansion in the bloodstream during pregnancy may prompt breakouts or skin inflammation. If you, as of now, have a skin break out the issue, it could turn out to be more terrible when you get pregnant. Even though skin breaks out doesn't represent any dangers to the pregnancy, you should be cautious when utilizing prescriptions or different items to avert or treat skin break out. To remain safe, counsel your primary care physician before attempting any therapeutic measures.

Cures:

- Don't utilize any rough skin items that may disturb your delicate skin.

- Some hostile to skin break out drugs may not be sheltered during pregnancy and ought to have stayed away from. Converse with your PCP before utilizing any drug.

• Mild face washes can be utilized to clean your face; however, check their fixings before use.

2. Skin labels

These are minor, free skin developments that may create during pregnancy. If you, as of now, have skin labels, they could duplicate when you get pregnant. They typically show up on the neck, close to the crotch region, and underarms. Skin labels are innocuous, and they carry no dangers to pregnancy.

Cures:

• You can go to the dermatologist and get them evacuated. The primary and speedy system may not require a sedative.

3. Stretch imprints

This could occur because of hormonal changes or extending your skin during pregnancy. Likewise named as striae gravidarum, stretch imprints can be seen in the stomach area, hindquarters, hips, and breasts. These imprints happen because of the extending of the elastic strands of the skin. These imprints are regular during pregnancy and will, in general, blur away after the delivery.

Cures:

• Moisturizing your skin with cocoa spread, olive oil, nutrient E cream, or aloe vera may help diminish stretch imprints.

• There are a couple of medications that should be possible baby blues too. These incorporate oral tretinoin treatment and laser treatment; however, there is constrained proof to demonstrate their adequacy. Consequently, you have to counsel a pro.

• You may likewise utilize some homegrown cures and stretch imprints expulsion creams that are ok for your skin. Be that as it may, counsel a specialist before having a go at anything.

4. Hyperpigmentation

This is usually a hormone-related skin condition. Around 90% of pregnant ladies could encounter pigmentation of specific zones of the skin, for example, the armpits, genital region, and areolas. This generally happens because pregnancy hormones trigger the generation of colors. Melasma and linea nigra are the two types of hyperpigmentation that pregnant ladies experience.

Cures:

• You may utilize sunscreen when going out, as UV beams can exacerbate the pigmentation. You could likewise take a couple of straightforward measures, for example, covering your skin and destroying a cap while going in the sun to diminish skin obscuring during and after pregnancy.

• Take a drug that incorporates Retin-A. After delivery, specialists may recommend creams that help blur the dull imprints.

5. Pruritic Urticarial Papules and Plaques of Pregnancy (PUPPP)

This pregnancy-explicit skin condition causes little red rashes or knocks, which are additionally irritated. It starts as a little ill-advised or knock on the mid-region and may form into a more magnificent fix later. The rash may likewise spread to the breasts, bottom, and thighs. Even though there are no unfriendly impacts of this on the pregnancy, getting it treated will assist you with dodging irritation and uneasiness.

Cures:

• Topical corticosteroids, oral antihistamines, and fundamental glucocorticoids are endorsed dependent on the seriousness of the rash.

• Oatmeal showers, wet and cold packs may give some alleviation from the irritation.

6. Prurigo of Pregnancy

Additionally, a pregnancy-explicit skin condition, this prompts little knocks, looking like creepy crawly nibbles on the skin. These are bothersome and could be brought about by invulnerability changes happening in the body. These keep going for quite a long time after the delivery also yet are not known to have any fetal dangers.

Cures:

• Cooling showers can give some help from irritation.

• Doctors endorse oral antihistamines and respectably strong topical steroids.

• Aqueous cream that contains menthol (1-2%) can likewise be applied whenever endorsed by the specialist.

7. Intrahepatic Cholestasis of Pregnancy (ICP)

This condition may create when the typical bile stream turns out to be moderate or quits during pregnancy. It causes itching, and sometimes may likewise bring about jaundice. ICP is generally experienced in the third trimester, though once in a while. There could be dangers of stillbirth, preterm birth, or fetal trouble. Henceforth, extreme itching ought not to be overlooked.

Cures:

• The board plan of ICP incorporates meds, early delivery, and fetal observing.

Drugs are endorsed dependent on the seriousness of the condition, fetal wellbeing, and gestational age.

8. Others

A couple of other, uncommon pregnancy-explicit skin conditions include:

• One in 50,000 pregnant ladies may encounter pemphigoid gestationis. Rarely, it could prompt unexpected labor. Else, it very well may be treated through meds.

• Impetigo herpetiformis is an uncommon pregnancy-explicit condition. There isn't a lot of research about this issue. Prescriptions could be given to treat the sores that it causes, yet the degree of hazard to the hatchling is obscure.

• Pruritic folliculitis of pregnancy, the etiology of this issue is questionable.

Would you be able to Prevent Skin Changes In Pregnancy?

You can't forestall yet can oversee them with therapeutic mediation and sometimes, regular or locally situated cures and topical creams. Healing estimates will help in controlling the rashes or irritation assuming any. Most skin changes experienced during pregnancy vanish after labor and are not usually a reason for concern. You may attempt simple to-utilize and safety measures to get the condition ward off the inconvenience. In any case, on the off chance that you imagine that the skin issue is disturbing you, you ought to get it checked by a specialist to counteract any confusion.

How To Reduce Breast Pain During Pregnancy

Before you appreciate the sweet moments of turning into a mother and make the most of your kid's first breath, there are certainly some mild pains you, as a to-be mother, may need to experience. It is guaranteeing to realize that it isn't merely you who are experiencing this, yet every mother out there who is sustaining her infant in the belly is confronting comparative highs and lows as you seem to be!

Why breast pain during pregnancy? Breast pain is truth to be told, one of the soonest potential pointers of pregnancy and isn't anomalous. It generally happens during the menstrual cycle for certain ladies; however, it is noticeably seen in the first three months during pregnancy. During this stage, your breasts feel delicately swollen, sore, or touchy. It begins from the fifth to sixth seven day stretch of the pregnancy. Yet, it is alleviating to realize that most ladies who are expecting a child see that the breast pain diminishes or nearly vanishes in the last 50% of their pregnancy.

Body type changes in ladies! Some are seen encountering persistent breast pain as long as they are conveying their child, while some others barely experience any pain at all. In this article, we present you probably the most widely recognized purposes behind which hopeful moms experience pain in the breast during pregnancy.

Regular Reasons Of Breast Pain In Pregnancy

1. Breast Changes which are Fibrocystic:

This is viewed as the most widely recognized reason for pain in the breast during pregnancy. In fibrocystic breast changes, small blisters structure in the fibrous tissue of the chest, get loaded up with liquid and swell, and lead to pain.

2. Awkwardness in the Hormone Levels:

During pregnancy, its characteristic is that the body sets itself up to experience numerous phases of the improvement of a child. This outcome in a fast change in various hormonal levels, especially an unevenness in the estrogen levels that generally brings about breast pain.

3. Breasts which Leak:

One of the most widely recognized grumblings from numerous hopeful moms is that their breasts break, and this is seen generally in the second or third trimester of pregnancy. Breast spills, for the most part, happen because your breasts start delivering colostrums. This is a thick-liquid that sustains your new-conceived infant in the first couple of days before your breasts start producing milk. This fluid is discharged from the chest because of a back rub or in any event when you are explicitly stimulated. It is one of the significant reasons for breast pain, particularly in the later phases of pregnancy. Utilizing a nursing cushion is a generally excellent solution for this issue.

4. Changes in the Breast:

The most significant capacity of your breasts is to nourish your child after delivery. Therefore, your breasts are bitten by a bit arranged by your body during the pregnancy time frame. During pregnancy, milk-creating cells and milk-pipes are shaped. This, in the long run, causes an expansion in the size of your breasts. It might be starting to realize that an ever-increasing number of layers of fat begin to amass underneath your breasts as you progress into your pregnancy arrange. Because of this, you will see an entirely unmistakable change in both the size and state of your breasts.

Shockingly, your breasts proceed with this procedure of developing to about a cup size in the underlying three months of maternity. These joined factors at last reason pain in the breast.

How To Reduce Breast Pain?

Since we have seen the different reasons and foundations for breast pain, let us look at how this pain can be handled! Here are some basic approaches to support you:

1. During your pregnancy, ensure you cautiously pick your inward articles of clothing, particularly your bra, to ensure that they bolster your breasts appropriately. Monitor your breast size as you may see massive changes, and as needs get another bra each time, you feel the requirement for one. A few people even wear more than one bra, if they think that one isn't adequate. Everything relies upon how agreeable you are. On the off chance that you abstain from wearing a bra, be prepared to confront the most exceedingly terrible pain, which at last influences your breast shape as well!

2. On the off chance that your breasts are excessively overwhelming or voluminous, take a stab at wearing games or a cushioned bra. They are commonly generally reasonable and agreeable for ladies with large breasts during pregnancy.

3. In all honesty, stopping on the admission of salt enormously helps in lessening the pain in your breasts. This is because salt holds water, because of which your breasts become heavier, bringing about intense pain.

4. Water is another mitigating choice. Do drink a lot of water during your whole pregnancy period. It aids in flushing out an abundance of waste liquids and also makes you feel lighter and fresher.

5. Ladies, for the most part, will, in general, take a ton of bed rest during and after pregnancy; however, the enchantment is being dynamic! It is critical to keep yourself physically energetic in little manners. They can be strolling for about thirty minutes day by day, doing some light family

unit errands, and so on. This will keep you dynamic by giving you decent blood flow and make you feel lighter.

6. Sometimes the pain might be too exceptional that nothing, unless there are other options safeguards may give help; for this situation, counsel your gynecologist for other healing measures. It is imperative to maintain a strategic distance from self-medicine to stay away from entanglements.

7. Ice cushions or warming cushions give solace to certain ladies. Before you use it consistently, test to perceive what suits you the best!

8. Exercises like reflection and yoga are said to keep the brain and body without a care in the world. This will, in the long run, help you in enduring breast pain during pregnancy.

Although, breast pain during pregnancy is humiliating, awkward, and painful, you ought to understand that it is typical and nothing to stress over. It a decent practice to continue counseling your gynecologist to guarantee that there are no difficulties related to this pregnancy indication.

Pregnancy is without a doubt, perhaps the most significant high in a lady's life and accompanies its very a lot of challenges too. On the off chance that you are hoping to anticipate your pregnancy, at that point, you should peruse this article and keep yourself rationally arranged to confront the circumstance. Once you do that, you won't be in such a shock after you get pregnant! Prepared to realize what are the adjustments in the body during pregnancy? At that point, read on.

Common Body Changes During Pregnancy

Here are some generally watched changes in the body during pregnancy that you can anticipate!

1. Sore Breasts:

The first indication of pregnancy is generally found on your breasts. They seem more significant, delicate, or even painful, on account of increased affectability. Such affectability can sometimes make you tense and awkward. Additionally, they won't get littler!

Prepare for more magnificent estimated breasts as you progress, starting with one trimester then onto the next. This is because the hormones are setting up your body to produce enough milk post-labor. There isn't a lot of you can do about it! Be glad for your measure and go out on the town to shop for greater ones, also the endorphins that shopping will give to keep us upbeat.

2. Mood Swings:

Mood swings are the most widely recognized physical changes during pregnancy. They are not new to ladies; we experience them at whatever point we have our cycles. Be that as it may, being pregnant is a severe deal to our body, so consider these as pre-menstrual strains on steroids! With the progression of hormones, you will be on a teeter-totter ride with feelings. Flooding your tear conduits given a chipped nail to crying containers while watching Finding Nemo is ordinary; have confidence, being a passionate wreck is a piece of the activity. Another component of mood-swing is the absurd hankering, frequently for abnormal mixes of nourishment! Enjoy, yet ensure your desires don't hurt your condition.

3. Morning Sickness:

As though being an anxious wreck was insufficient, here comes the disgusting morning infection. Some even wind up retching more often than not in spite of the cures set up. It occurs in the first trimester, where one feels like there are on a three-month-long headache! There is a unique advantage for certain ladies who don't get morning ailment by any stretch of the imagination. This is marginally out of line for the other people who need to endure genuinely. However, then it stops nearly all of a sudden, so don't stress over it.

4. Skin Conditions:

While it is a typical idea that ladies gleam during pregnancy, it isn't valid for all ladies. Because of the hormone surge, some expecting moms may have immense episodes of skin inflammation, rashes, and pigmentation all over. This can likewise be seen on the neck and breasts. These are child flushes that don't as well, frenzy and hurry to the ER. When the child shows up, mommy will improve the skin. Another effect on the surface is the presence of stretch imprints. You will explode to twice your size during pregnancy, so clearly, you may discover stretch imprints, for the most part, around the stomach district. Utilize a Vitamin E rich body oil to keep them negligible.

5. Liquid Retention:

The body begins holding more liquids during pregnancy and may prompt swollen lower legs, puffy face, and swollen fingers. It deteriorates during summers, which is the reason for staying away from sodium (salt), and even sugar is a decent beginning stage. Drink loads of water, since that causes you to flush the salt out. Water maintenance requires the specialist's consideration so ensure you have legitimate subsequent meet-ups with your doctor.

6. Weight Gain:

Indeed, pregnancy is a time when we put on the most extreme load to oblige the child. However, it very well may be a success at your confidence. Add to that the raging hormones, and you wind up feeling tragic and discouraged. A decent and adoring condition guarantees that the mythical pregnancy shine originates from inside. At the point when I state it's not beautiful, I mean the noticeable protruding veins on your legs and vulva because of the abundance weight. Be cautious about these and attempt to have them concealed to abstain from feeling less appealing. Moms must be in a decent mental plane consistently, as it guarantees a solid and cheerful mother and infant baby blues.

7. Hyperactive Bladder:

Expanded pee during pregnancy is normal. While the infant moves around in the belly, the moms feel the kick over their bladder. Sometimes you won't arrive at the loo on time! Be that as it may, you will make the excursion in any event 20 times a day. Doing pelvic floor exercises is a decent method to guarantee that you don't feel overworked. Also, indeed, by all means, drink heaps of water since it is fundamental to pee as you need its capacity to flush the poisons out of your body.

8. Solid discharges:

Obstruction is likewise one of the regular body changes in pregnancy, particularly on the off chance that you are on iron enhancements. The ideal approach to maintain a strategic distance from this is by taking iron-rich nourishments and not supplements. Have natural products like banana, apples, and veggies like spinach or any greens. They were altogether made by Mother Nature for our needs. As they state, moms consistently know best.

9. Heartburn/Indigestion:

Indigestion or heartburn and acid reflux can be painful during pregnancy. While the child develops in the belly, it gets your organs squished up, attempting to make its space. This makes you awkward after eating as a result of this constrained confinement. The best arrangement is to eat littler dinners often. One can likewise depend on home-prepared teas for help.

10. Changes in Sex Life:

Hormonal changes can make you need either pretty much of sex. Both the circumstances are conceivable, in light of the condition of hormones. Any attempt to get a parity much as could reasonably be expected and see what works out. This might be the most you can get continuous before your kid begins going to class!

How To Stop Snoring During Pregnancy

Pregnant ladies are probably going to gasp, particularly in the third trimester. Research expresses that 35% of ladies report snoring each day or three to four times per week. 26% wheeze during pregnancy.

Is Snoring Common During Pregnancy?

Snoring during pregnancy is moderately healthy, particularly in the third trimester. Concentrates likewise uncover that constant snoring (three to more evenings in seven days) increments from 7% to 11% in the first trimester and 16% to 25% in the third trimester. Snoring could be innocuous the more significant part of the times, however now and again, it could show a hidden condition that could be destructive to you or the infant. Comprehending what causes snoring is fundamental to handle it the correct way.

What Are The Causes Of Snoring During Pregnancy?

The following are the potential reasons for snoring during pregnancy.

1. Nasal clog: The expanding estrogen levels during pregnancy bring about the growth of the mucous layer along the nasal sections. It builds the creation of bodily fluid, prompting clog in the nasal pit and at last snoring. Additionally, an expansion in the blood volume grows the veins, causing an expanding of the nasal films. This makes breathing troublesome and may bring about snoring.

2. Fatigue: You may feel incredibly drained when you are pregnant. This will prompt a profound sleep, during which you will lose power over the throat muscles. The muscles become excessively loose and deter the aviation routes, causing vibrations as you inhale, making the snoring sound.

3. Weight addition: The expanding weight during pregnancy adds some additional fat to your neck and throat districts too. This other tissue packs the aviation routes, makes breathing troublesome and causes snoring.

4. Sleep apnea: Loud snoring could be one of the side effects of obstructive rest apnea (OSA). It is where you quit breathing suddenly during rest, because of a blockage in the aviation routes. OSA has different manifestations, for example, heaving commotions and daytime languor.

5. Colds and hypersensitivities: Cold, influenza, or sensitivities will likewise prompt snoring since they bring about nasal clog, which makes breathing troublesome.

Snoring during pregnancy could be a transitory condition, caused because of the adjustments in the body. In any case, that isn't the situation consistently.

Are There Any Complications Associated With Snoring During Pregnancy?

Snoring may not be a reason for concern. Be that as it may, on the off chance that it is, you should realize how to distinguish it and look for therapeutic intercession.

Concentrates by the University of Michigan and the Northwestern University Feinberg School of Medicine express that snoring could demonstrate a hazard for the mother and the infant in the accompanying cases.

• The swollen veins, because of a nasal clog or weight gain, will limit the progression of blood to the placenta, denying the infant of supplements and blood.

• Habitual snoring is related to poor results for both the mom and the infant, including the danger of cesarean segment and low birth weight babies.

• Frequent snoring is probably going to cause gestational diabetes, which could build the danger of type 2 diabetes later in life.

• There is a greater danger of preeclampsia because of unreasonable snoring during pregnancy, which could prompt premature labor and fatalities.

• Another difficulty may be intrauterine development confinement (IUGR) that causes littler children with formative postponements.

On the off chance that snoring is because of a fundamental ailment, at that point, treating the condition will stop the snoring too. If it is because of the substantial changes during pregnancy, you can attempt the cures we let you know straight away.

How To Stop Snoring When Pregnant?

You may attempt these straightforward solutions for overseeing snoring.

1. Use nasal splashes or strips that are promptly accessible in drug stores, and are a medication-free approach to oversee snoring. They clear the obstacle of the nasal sections and avert snoring.

2. Use a warm-fog humidifier in your room to treat your nasal clog and get help from snoring. Pick a humidifier that labors for eight hours or more for undisturbed rest.

3. Sleep on your left side to improve the blood course, and rest sufficiently.

4. Elevate your head within any event two cushions to permit the free progression of air. This will ease breathing and lessen snoring.

5. Watch your dietary patterns to abstain from gathering a higher number of calories than required. Overabundance weight addition could be one reason for snoring. In this way, watch what you eat and keep away from nourishments with zero nutritional worth.

6. Quit smoking, liquor, and sleeping pills as they can hinder the aviation routes and result in snoring. They are additionally dangerous for both the pregnant mom and the infant.

On the off chance that these cures don't help and your snoring is making you awkward, you have to visit the specialist.

When Should You See A Doctor?

If you are snoring more than expected, educate your primary care physician regarding it. Likewise, call the specialist on the off chance that you have the indications of preeclampsia.

• Daytime drowsiness

• A cerebral pain that will not leave

• Swollen legs

Preeclampsia is a crisis. Much of the time, a conclusion of preeclampsia will require early delivery.

When Will Snoring Go Away?

You are probably going to quit snoring in the wake of conveying the infant. If not quick, you will dispose of it after pregnancy, as you lose the child's weight.

Do Pregnant Women Snore More Than Others?

Indeed, pregnant ladies are probably going to pant more than non-pregnant ladies due to their expanding estrogen levels, belly, and blood dissemination. The individuals who never gasped pregnancy may build up the condition during pregnancy. Fortunately, you won't gasp until the end of time. When your child is here, the snoring is destined to disappear. Yet, restless evenings? They are digging in for the long haul for some time! Expect to discover your accomplice insightfully discussing those delightful 'wheeze filled' evenings!

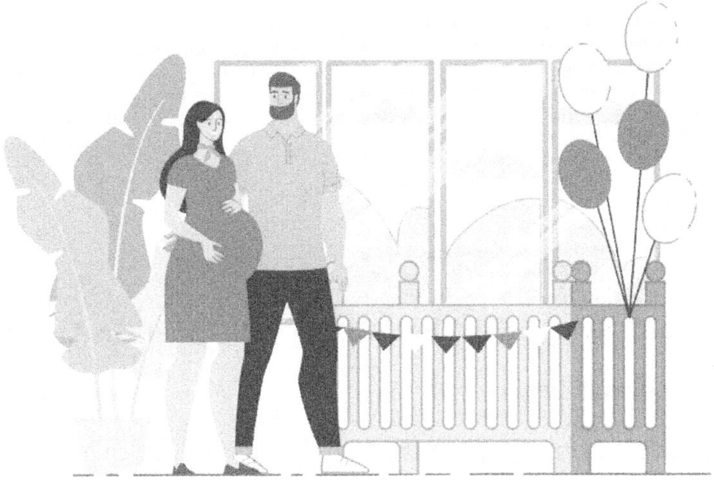

"Truthfully, being pregnant is changing me as a person. Each day is part of this amazing journey that has completely shifted the focus of my life and made me reevaluate my personal and professional goals." *– Holly Madison*

"Pregnancy is a process that invites you to surrender to the unseen force behind all life." *– Judy Ford*

CHAPTER FIVE

IMPORTANT PIECES THAT ALL FIRST-TIME MOMS MUST KNOW

Realities About Newborns That All Parents Must Be Aware Of

1. He looks somewhat clever

A long way from the photos of tubby infants you're accustomed to seeing on each magazine spread, site, and handout you've perused all through your pregnancy, your infant's looks may come as an amazement.

He'll be very red and wrinkly and may even game an excellent covering of hair over his body called "lanugo" (this will leave after some time). What's more, on the off chance that you had a vaginal birth, his face may look somewhat squashed. He'll smooth out soon enough, however.

2. The first crap will shock you

For the first not many days, your child's stools comprise of meconium, a clingy greenish dark substance that lined your infant's digestion tracts during pregnancy. To tidy it up, wipe your infant's base with a chunk of cotton fleece plunged in the water and coat your infant's bottom in oil jam, so it's simpler to expel whenever.

3. He will be ravenous

Try not to be convinced to give your infant oat in his jug by good-natured family "to assist him with feeling full" – your child is going to require a feed each a few hours and beginning him on solids early is exceptionally hazardous.

"After birth, your infant will require sustenance to develop and create, and since his belly is still tiny, he will take in enough nutrition to see him through only a couple of hours before requiring another feed," says child master and coauthor of Sleep Sense Meg Faure.

4. He won't stay asleep for the entire evening

Honestly, your new infant will rest a ton. Be that as it may, he'll additionally awaken a ton. "Infants will wake around evening time as much as they do during the day for nutritional reasons. The infant has been accustomed to having nutrition 'on tap,'" says Meg. Anticipate that your infant should wake up as frequently as each a few hours in these early days to encourage.

5. He can't see far

For the first scarcely any long stretches of his life, your child can concentrate on objects 20 to 30 cm before him. This energizes your holding as it's just about the precise separation between his face and yours while you feed him.

6. You don't need to shower him consistently

Since your infant won't do much in these early days (and because that infant skin is so fragile), you won't have to do a full shower each day. A quick wipe down of the significant bits is all you have to keep him clean. This is called top and following – where you utilize a bit of clammy cotton fleece (plunged in cooled, bubbled water) to wipe your endearing face's, bum territory, arms, and overlays of skin. Utilize another bit of cotton fleece for each piece of the body.

7. Continuously go aroma free

If you choose to shower your child, make sure to utilize infant items that are free of any scents. That infant skin isn't accustomed to being out on the planet yet, and the exact opposite thing you need to do is aggravate it.

8. He is loud!

For such a minor thing, your infant can make a dangerous racket. Other than the crying, he'll be snorting, moaning, grunting, and then some. Babies' nasal entries are still very restricted, and caught bodily fluid prompts some entirely peculiar audio effects on occasion. Get his nose out with a decent saline shower. Infants additionally wheeze a great deal.

9. You may not experience passionate feelings for him immediately

In the wake of nine monotonous months of pregnancy, you may expect the moment you first meet your child to top you off with moment and intense adoration. Be that as it may, for certain moms, it doesn't occur along these lines, and that is ordinary.

Holding can take some time – recollect that much like pregnancy and labor, it is distinctive for everybody. There's no correct path for clinging to occur, so give it time. On the off chance that regardless you feel along these lines following half a month, or you have negative emotions towards your child, make sure to converse with your primary care physician to preclude postnatal gloom.

10. His skin may strip

In the wake of coasting around in a pool of "water" for a long while, your child's introduction to dry air can play destruction with his delicate skin. Around his second or third day, you may see his skin become flaky as it acclimates to life outside the belly. This will amend in a brief span.

11. He won't make a crap each day

It's essential for infants to pass stool as regularly as seven times per day, or as rarely as once in seven days. What's more, he'll snort and moan as he's creation that crap. This is ordinary and doesn't mean your infant has the runs or is blocked up. For whatever length of time that your child is encouraging excellent and wetting his nappy regularly, there's nothing to stress over.

12. He will cry, a ton

Crying is your child's method for speaking with you, so anticipate a ton of it. At first, this will be somewhat overpowering, mainly as he'll cry when he's hungry, hot or chilly, worn out, feeling forlorn, and the sky is the limit from there. Sooner or later, you'll make sense of how to react to every sort of cry. Until further notice, however, it's experimentation.

13. He could have boobs

While somewhat unsettling, swollen privates and even the presence of breasts is typical. Those hormones that tormented you all through pregnancy additionally affect your infant, and these will vanish following half a month. You may likewise see a pink release in your daughter's nappy for a similar explanation.

14. You basically can't ruin him

Your infant needs to feel cherished and secure, and his crying isn't an approach to be devious. Hold him regularly, snuggle and converse with him, feed him on request and react to all his cries. You are not ruining him, however, setting down establishments for a solid bond.

15. Leave that stump from that umbilical rope alone!

It's one of the nastier pieces of infant child-rearing, and you most likely can hardly wait for that unattractive umbilical string stump to leave. Be that as it may, pulling on it trying to hustle the procedure along is just going to drag out it, and can even wind up in disease. The ideal approach to urge that stump to tumble off is to keep it dry.

16. His eye shading will change

All infants are brought into the world with dim blue eyes and change to their genuine nature with time. What shading his eyes will choose genuinely relies upon the measure of melanin in the iris. You'll see the most dramatic change in eye shading somewhere in the range of six and nine months, so get your fill of that postnatal depression while you can!

17. He should invest energy in his belly

Belly time is an unquestionable requirement, in any event, for minor infants. "Babies ought to invest energy in their bellies to fortify their back muscles. The first gross engine task a child has is to uncurl and build up his back muscles, and the ideal approach to do this is by guaranteeing he has some belly time when wakeful. Infants ought not, nonetheless, rest on their bellies.

18. He can recognize you by the smell

Your child's feeling of smell created in the belly, and thus it's probably the most grounded sense present during childbirth. Truth be told, your infant's perception of smell will assist him with distinguishing you, as he can perceive your aroma when he's seven days old. This is another way that nature guarantees an extraordinary bond between you.

19. He is diverse to a "child infant."

Babies don't do a lot, honestly. For the first month and a half, you'll be kept so occupied by your little group. However, all he'll truly be doing is sleeping, crying, drinking milk, crapping, and sleeping, crying, drinking, and crapping some more. It might feel similar to an unpleasant activity, yet once the child spends the six-week point and "awakens" a little, you can anticipate coos, sputters, and more significant action.

20. It goes rapidly

While it is the most troublesome thing you've at any point done in your life, this intensive lesson in child-upbringing is a brilliant time. Before long, you'll be getting more rest and feel more yourself. Be that as it may, you won't have these first hardly any days with your child until the end of time, so attempt to appreciate it – in one way or another.

What's in store During a Vaginal Delivery

Picking a vaginal delivery

Each delivery is as novel and individual as each mother and newborn child. Likewise, ladies may have various encounters with each new labor and delivery. Conceiving an offspring is a groundbreaking occasion that will leave an impact on you for a fantastic remainder. You'll need this to be a positive encounter and to recognize what's in store. Here's some data about what may occur as you're conveying your child.

Birth plans: Should you have one?

As you approach the last piece of your pregnancy, you might need to compose a birth plan. Consider cautiously what's essential to you. The general objective is a solid mother and child. The birth plan diagrams your optimal birth and may be balanced as the real circumstance unfurls. Chat with your accomplice and choose who you need to have to go to the delivery. A few couples feel this is a private time and favor not to have others present. A birth plan may incorporate different subjects like pain alleviation during labor, delivery positions, and the sky is the limit from there.

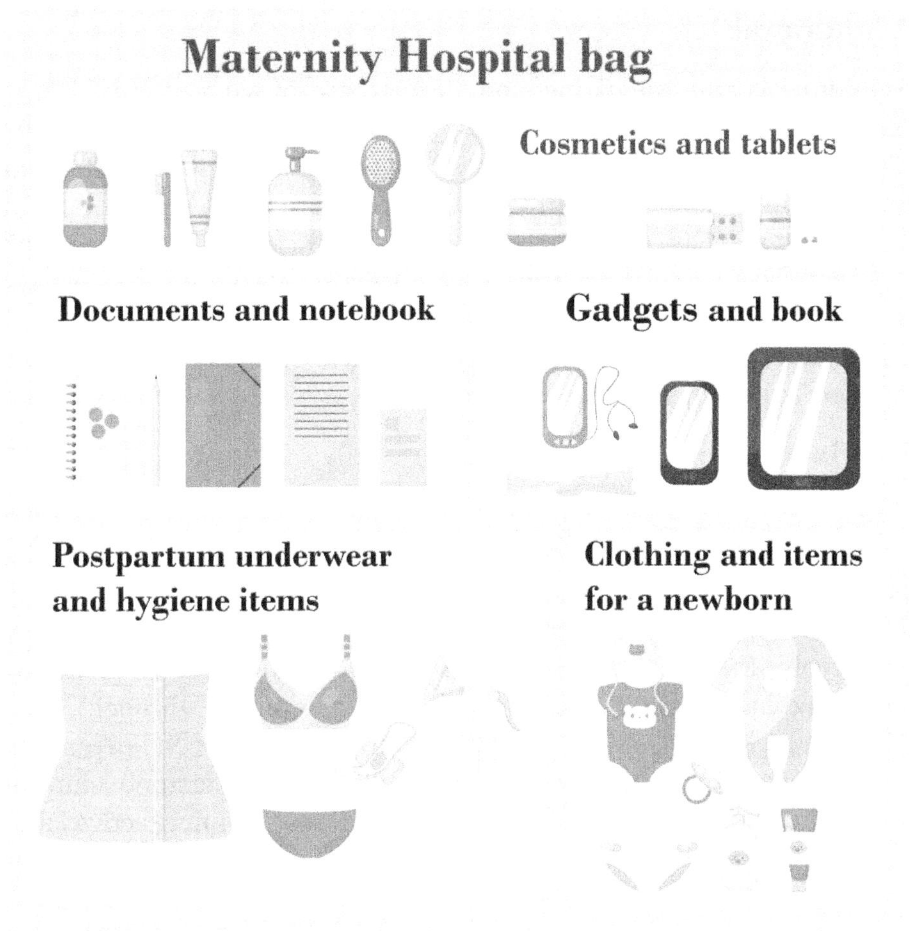

Early periods of labor

Amniotic sac

The amniotic sac is the liquid-filled layer encompassing your child. This sac will quite often break before the infant is conceived; however, sometimes, it stays flawless until delivery. At the point when it cracks, it's frequently portrayed as your "water breaking." In many cases, your water will break before you start giving birth or at the earliest reference point of labor. Most ladies experience their water breaking as a spout of liquid. It ought to be clear and unscented — if it's yellow, green, or dark-colored, contact your primary care physician immediately.

Withdrawals

Withdrawals are the fixing and discharging of your uterus. These movements will, in the long run, help your child push through the cervix. Constrictions can feel like substantial squeezing or weight that starts in your back and moves to the front. Compressions aren't a solid pointer of labor. You may, as of now, have felt Braxton-Hicks withdrawals, which may have begun as right on time as your subsequent trimester. A general guideline is that when you have constrictions that keep going for a moment, are five minutes separated, and have been so for 60 minutes, and you're in evident labor.

Cervix widening

The cervix is the most reduced piece of the uterus that opens into the vagina. The cervix is a rounded structure around 3 to 4 centimeters long with an entry that interfaces the uterine cavity to the vagina. During labor, the job of the cervix must change from keeping up the pregnancy (by keeping the uterus shut) to encouraging the delivery of the infant (by widening or opening, enough to permit the infant through). The fundamental changes that happen close to the finish of the pregnancy bring about the conditioning of the cervical tissue and the diminishing of the cervix, the two of which help set up the uterus. Genuine, active labor is viewed as in progress when the cervix is enlarged 3 centimeters or more.

Labor and delivery

In the long run, the cervical trench must open until the cervical opening itself has arrived at 10 centimeters in the distance across, and the child can go into the birth waterway. As the infant enters the vagina, your skin and muscles stretch. The labia and perineum (the zone between the vagina and the rectum) in the end arrive at a point of most extreme extending. Now, the skin may feel like its consuming. Some labor instructors call this the ring of fire as a result of the consuming sensation felt as the mother's tissues stretch around the child's head. As of now, your human services supplier may choose to play out an episiotomy. You might feel the episiotomy because the skin and muscles can lose sensation because of how firmly they're extended.

The birth

As the infant's head develops, there is an incredible alleviation from the weight, even though you'll likely still feel some uneasiness. Your medical caretaker or specialist will request that you quit pushing momentarily while the child's mouth and nose are suctioned to get out the amniotic liquid and bodily fluid. It's imperative to do this before the child begins to inhale and cry. Generally, the specialist will pivot the child's head a fourth of a go-to be in arrangement with the infant's body, which is still inside you. You'll, at that point, be approached to start pushing again to convey the shoulders. The top shoulder starts things out and, afterward, the lower joint. At that point, with one final push, you send your infant!

Conveying the placenta

The placenta and the amniotic sac that bolstered and ensured the child for nine months are still in the uterus after the delivery. These should be conveyed, and this can happen suddenly, or it might take as long as thirty minutes. Your birthing assistant or specialist may rub your belly beneath your belly catch to help fix the uterus and slacken the placenta. Your uterus is presently about the size of a large grapefruit. You may need to push to help convey the placenta. You may feel some weight as the placenta is removed, however, not so much pressure as when the infant was conceived.

Your social insurance supplier will investigate the conveyed placenta to ensure it was sent in full. On uncommon events, a portion of the placenta doesn't discharge and may remain clung to the mass of the uterus. In the fact that this occurs, your supplier will venture into your uterus to evacuate the remaining pieces to counteract substantial draining that can result from a torn placenta. In the event that you might want to see the placenta, it would be ideal if you inquire. As a rule, they'll be glad to show you.

Pain and different sensations during delivery

When you choose a characteristic labor

If you choose to have characteristic labor (delivery without pain medicine), you'll feel a wide range of sensations. The two impressions you'll encounter the most are pain and weight. At the point when you start to push, a portion of the pressure will be soothed. As the infant plunges into the birth trench, however, you'll go from encountering constrain just during the constrictions to facing consistent and expanding pressure. It will feel something like a compelling impulse to have a stable discharge as the infant pushes down on those equivalent nerves.

If you decide to have an epidural

On the off chance that you have an epidural, what you feel during labor will rely upon the adequacy of the epidural square. On the off chance that the drug appropriately stifles the nerves, you may not feel anything. On the off chance that it's decently compelling, you may feel some weight. On the off chance that it's gently in this way, you'll feel the pressure that could be awkward to you. It relies upon how well you endure pressure sensations. You may not feel the extending of the vagina, and you likely won't feel an episiotomy.

Conceivable tearing

Albeit noteworthy wounds aren't healthy, during the enlargement procedure, the cervix may tear and eventually require a fix. Vaginal tissues are delicate and adaptable. However, if delivery happens quickly or with unnecessary power, those tissues can tear. By and large, slashes are minor and effectively fixed. Sometimes, they might be progressively genuine and bring about longer-term issues. Ordinary labor and delivery regularly bring about damage to the vagina and additionally cervix. Up to 70 percent of ladies having their first child will have an episiotomy or some vaginal tear requiring a fix. Luckily, the vagina and cervix have an abundant blood supply. That is the reason wounds in these regions mend rapidly and leave practically zero scarring that could bring about long-haul issues.

It's not difficult to set yourself up for labor and delivery, yet it's a broadly flighty procedure. Understanding the timeline and catching wind of other moms' encounters can go far to making labor less strange. Numerous eager moms think that it's accommodating to work out a birth plan with their accomplice and offer it with their therapeutic group. If you do make an arrangement, be set up to alter your perspective if the need emerges. Recollect that you will probably have a substantial child and a sound, positive encounter.

HOW WAS MY LABOUR AND DELIVERY?

Where, when and how the labour happened? ____________________

____

____

Which position you choose for delivery? ______________________

____

Was it painful?____

____

Additional notes to remember: _________________________________

____

____

Vote for myself: __________ Vote for my boyfriend: ____________

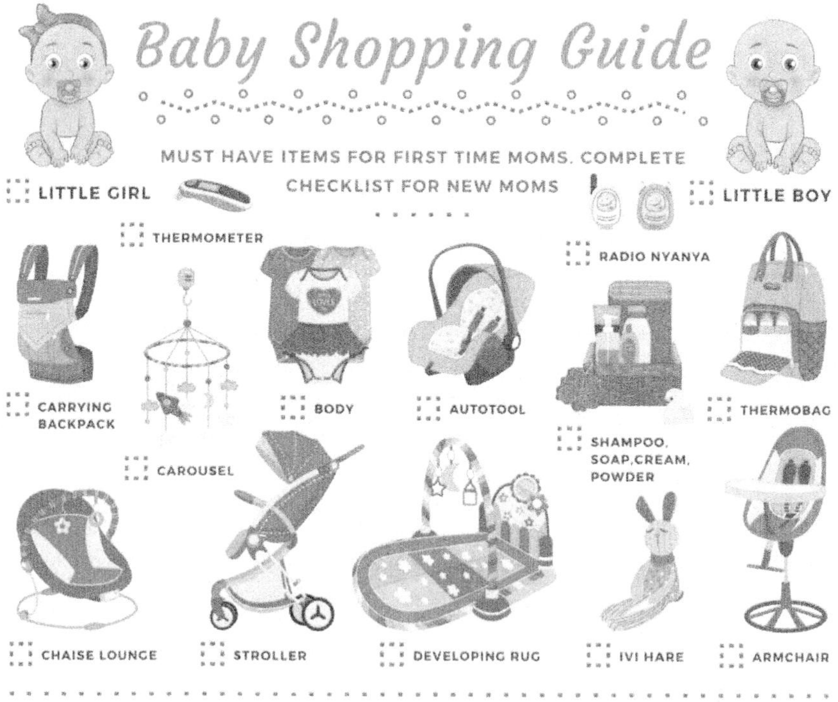
Baby Shopping Guide
MUST HAVE ITEMS FOR FIRST TIME MOMS. COMPLETE CHECKLIST FOR NEW MOMS
LITTLE GIRL
THERMOMETER
LITTLE BOY
RADIO NYANYA
CARRYING BACKPACK
CAROUSEL
BODY
AUTOTOOL
THERMOBAG
SHAMPOO, SOAP,CREAM, POWDER
CHAISE LOUNGE
STROLLER
DEVELOPING RUG
IVI HARE
ARMCHAIR

HAPPY MOTHERHOOD!